1991

Gift of Life

Catholic Scholars
Respond to the
Vatican Instruction

Gift of Life

Catholic Scholars
Respond to the
Vatican Instruction

Edmund D. Pellegrino
John Collins Harvey
John P. Langan
Editors

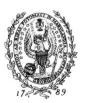

GEORGETOWN UNIVERSITY PRESS
Washington, D.C.

Library of Congress Cataloging-in-Publication Data

Gift of life : Catholic scholars respond to the Vatican Instruction /
   edited by E.D. Pellegrino, John Collins Harvey, and John P. Langan
   with the assistance of V.A. Sharpe.
       p.   cm.
   Papers presented at a conference sponsored by Georgetown
University.
   Includes English translation of: Donum vitae
   ISBN 0-87840-499-6
   1. Human reproductive technology--Religious aspects--Catholic
Church--Congresses.   2. Catholic Church. Congregatio pro Doctrina
Fidei.   Donum vitae--Congresses.   3. Catholic Church--Doctrines-
-Congresses.   I. Pellegrino, Edmund D., 1920-   . II. Harvey, John
Collins.   III. Langan, John, 1940-   . IV. Sharpe, V.A.
V. Georgetown University.   VI. Catholic Church.   Congregatio pro
Doctrina Fidei.   Donum vitae.   English.   1990.
RG133.5.G54   1990
176--dc20   90-30838
                                                                      CIP

Contents

Preface

It is a truism that ours is the "Age of Biology"—the era in which humans first asserted control over the processes of life. In our time, the beginnings and ends of human life, the fabric of its heredity, disease and behavior, and the fate of the species itself have become susceptible to exploration and manipulation. The previously sacred precincts of procreation, the family and of love itself have become the domain of molecular biology. What lags behind is the response to the unprecedented moral dilemmas which the wise use of our new biologic knowledge must entail.

The moral responses have largely been of two kinds—secular and religious. Those who do not believe in an objective moral order outside the human will have taken a utilitarian stance. Why not exploit nature's laws fully so long as the final sum of good done outweighs the harms and dangers? Do not the benefits of the eradication of disease, suffering, or unwanted or defective children, and the chance to reshape the human species override antiquated cultural and religious beliefs? Is it morally defensible not to exploit what we know?

Believers in a creator, in a natural and divine law governing human existence are divided in their responses. Fundamentalists decry "playing God" and forbid any interventions into life processes. The more liberal of the believers, on the other hand, urge us to join God as "co-creators" and help reshape human destiny since God himself is in "process." The Roman Catholic tradition has in general always taken a more balanced stance—fostering the advance of human knowledge, yet insisting that science and technology must always be under the constraint of the moral norms inscribed in divine and natural laws.

This is the spirit in which the now famous Vatican Instruction was presented in 1987. In this document, entitled *The*

Instruction on Respect for Human Life in its Origin and on the Dignity of Procreation, the Sacred Congregation for the Doctrine of the Faith confronts the moral dilemmas inherent in the newer reproductive technologies. Asserting the Catholic moral tradition with respect to procreation of human life, marriage and the dignity of the human person, the Instruction acknowledges the importance of the research and use of biological knowledge while defining the moral perimeters within which that knowledge may legitimately be used.

The Instruction also recognizes the urgency and complexity of the issues and invites the response of all Catholics to its statement. This is the invitation to which the scholars in this volume have responded. The papers presented here were delivered at Georgetown University at a conference of invited scholars, experts in ethics and in the reproductive technology in question. Professors Damewood and Huber, who are physicians, provided the technical background on the use of reproductive technologies such as in vitro fertilization. Theologians Cahill, Schüller, Haas and Sgreccia discuss the moral implications. Archbishop Quinn and Dean Frankino, a churchman and legal scholar, comment from the standpoint of American political philosophy on the document's exhortation to Catholics to participate in shaping laws and statutes in accordance with Roman Catholic moral teaching. The three editors of this volume—John Langan, S.J., John C. Harvey, and Edmund D. Pellegrino—provide commentaries for the sessions they chaired.

When the Instruction first appeared, the responses were immediate. Some were critical, some complimentary, some emotional and some restrained. The degree of interest within and outside the church spoke to the immediacy of the issues for many people. Responses were often conditioned on prior commitments for, or against, in vitro fertilization. This is unfortunate because much of the substance of the document was lost in debate over in vitro fertilization, which was but one part of a very substantial and fundamental disquisition on the moral dimensions of biology in human affairs. In some cases, secular commentators understood more clearly the positive dimensions of the Instruction than did some Roman Catholics themselves.

The papers in this volume have some advantages over the more immediate debates. They enjoy the distance of time from publication of the document. They were prepared after deliberation. They had the benefit of discussion by the other participants. Each author was afforded the subsequent opportunity to modify, clarify, emend and amend her/his remarks.

Readers will find differences of viewpoint in the section dealing with the moral-theological implications of the document. These differences reflect debate within the church itself. Given the moral sensitivity of the issues, their newness and the rapidity with which biological knowledge changes, divergence of opinion should not be surprising. The authors are committed Roman Catholics who take seriously the Sacred Congregation's invitation to respond to its pronouncement. It is in the spirit of faithful and conscientious commitment to the Roman Catholic moral tradition that these essays are offered.

The organizing committee wishes to acknowledge the encouragement and support of the Rev. Timothy S. Healy, S.J. Father Healy originated the idea for this conference as the proper way for a Catholic university to respond to the invitation of the Sacred Congregation for reflections on its Instruction. It also seemed fitting to include these considerations among the other publications marking the Bicentennial of Georgetown University.

Contributors

LISA SOWLE CAHILL, Ph.D. is Associate Professor in the Department of Theology, Boston College, Chestnut Hill, Massachusetts.

MARIAN D. DAMEWOOD, M.D. is Assistant Professor of Ob/Gyn and Director of the In Vitro Fertilization Program at Johns Hopkins Hospital, Baltimore, Maryland.

STEPHEN P. FRANKINO, J.D. is Dean of the School of Law, Villanova University, Villanova, Pennsylvania.

JOHN HAAS, Ph.D. is Assistant Professor of Theology at the Pontifical College Josephinum, Columbus, Ohio.

JOHN COLLINS HARVEY, M.D., Ph.D. is Professor of Medicine Emeritus at the Georgetown University Medical Center and a Senior Research Scholar at the Kennedy Institute of Ethics, Georgetown University, Washington, D.C.

JOHANNES HUBER is Dozent in Ob/Gyn at the University of Vienna and Director of the In Vitro Fertilization Program at the Allgemeines Krankenhaus, Vienna, Austria.

JOHN P. LANGAN, S.J. is the Rose F. Kennedy Professor of Christian Ethics at the Kennedy Institute of Ethics and a Senior Research Fellow at the Woodstock Theological Center, Georgetown University, Washington, D.C.

EDMUND D. PELLEGRINO, M.D. is the Director of the Georgetown University Center for the Advanced Study of Ethics and the John Carroll Professor of Medicine and Medical Humanities at Georgetown University, Washington, D.C.

MOST REV. JOHN R. QUINN, D.D. is the Archbishop of San Francisco, California.

BRUNO SCHÜLLER, S.J. is Professor of Moral Philosophy at Westfalische Wilhelms-Universität, Münster, West Germany.

MSGR. ELIO SGRECCIA is Director of the Centro di Bioetica Facoltà di Medicina di Chirurgia, Rome, Italy.

I.

INSTRUCTION ON RESPECT FOR HUMAN LIFE IN ITS ORIGIN AND ON THE DIGNITY OF PROCREATION

REPLIES TO CERTAIN QUESTIONS OF THE DAY

Issued by the
Congregation for the Doctrine of the Faith

Foreword

The Congregation for the Doctrine of the Faith has been approached by various episcopal conferences or individual bishops, by theologians, doctors and scientists, concerning biomedical techniques which make it possible to intervene in the initial phase of the life of a human being and in the very processes of procreation and their conformity with the principles of Catholic morality. The present Instruction, which is the result of wide consultation and in particular of a careful evaluation of the declarations made by episcopates, does not intend to repeat all the church's teaching on the dignity of human life as it originates and on procreation, but to offer, in the light of the previous teaching of the magisterium, some specific replies to the main questions being asked in this regard.

The exposition is arranged as follows: an *introduction* will recall the fundamental principles, of an anthropological and moral character, which are necessary for a proper evaluation of the problems and for working out replies to those questions; the *first part* will have as its subject respect for the human being from the first moment of his or her existence; the *second part* will deal with the moral questions raised by technical interventions on human procreation; the *third part* will offer some orientations on the relationships between moral law and civil law in terms of the respect due to human embryos and fetuses* and as regards the legitimacy of techniques of artificial procreation.

---

* The terms "zygote," "pre-embryo," "embryo," and "fetus" can indicate in the vocabulary of biology successive states of the development of a human being. The present Instruction makes free use of these terms, attributing to them an identical ethical relevance, in order to designate the result (whether visible or not) of human generation, from the first moment of its existence until birth. The reason for this usage is clarified by the text (cf. I, 1).

INTRODUCTION

1. Biomedical Research and the Teaching of the Church

The gift of life which God the Creator and Father has entrusted to man calls him to appreciate the inestimable value of what he has been given and to take responsibility for it: this fundamental principle must be placed at the center of one's reflection in order to clarify and solve the moral problems raised by artificial interventions on life as it originates and on the processes of procreation.

Thanks to the progress of the biological and medical sciences, man has at his disposal ever more effective therapeutic resources; but he can also acquire new powers, with unforeseeable consequences, over human life at its very beginning and in its first stages. Various procedures now make it possible to intervene not only in order to assist but also to dominate the processes of procreation. These techniques can enable man to "take in hand his own destiny," but they also expose him "to the temptation to go beyond the limits of a reasonable dominion over nature."[1] They might constitute progress in the service of man, but they also involve serious risks. Many people are therefore expressing an urgent appeal that in interventions on procreation the values and rights of the human person be safeguarded. Requests for clarification and guidance are coming not only from the faithful but also from those who recognize the church as "an expert in humanity"[2] with a mission to serve the "civilization of love"[3] and of life.

The church's magisterium does not intervene on the basis of a particular competence in the area of the experimental sciences; but having taken account of the data of research and technology, it intends to put forward, by virtue of its evangelical mission and apostolic duty, the moral teaching corresponding to the dignity of the person and to his or her integral vocation. It intends to do so by expounding the criteria of moral judgment as regards the applications of scientific research and technology, especially in relation to human life and its beginnings. These criteria are the respect, defense and promotion of man, his "primary and fundamental right" to life,[4] his dignity as a person endowed with a spiritual soul and moral responsibility,[5] and called to beatific communion with God.

The church's intervention in this field is inspired also by the love which she owes to man, helping him to recognize and respect his rights and duties. This love draws from the fount of Christ's love: as she contemplates the mystery of the Incarnate Word, the church also comes to understand the "mystery of man";[6] by proclaiming the Gospel of salvation, she reveals to man his dignity and invites him to discover fully the truth of his own being. Thus the church once more puts forward the divine law in order to accomplish the work of truth and liberation.

For it is out of goodness—in order to indicate the path of life—that God gives human beings his commandments and the grace to observe them: and it is likewise out of goodness—in order to help them persevere along the same path—that God always offers to everyone his forgiveness. Christ has compassion on our weaknesses: he is our Creator and Redeemer. May his spirit open men's hearts to the gift of God's peace and to an understanding of his precepts.

2. Science and Technology
at the Service of the Human Person

God created man in his own image and likeness: "male and female he created them" (Gn 1:27), entrusting to them the task of "having dominion over the earth" (Gn 1:28). Basic scientific research and applied research constitute a significant expression of this dominion of man over creation. Science and technology are valuable resources for man when placed at his service and when they promote his integral development for the benefit of all; but they cannot of themselves show the meaning of existence and of human progress. Being ordered to man, who initiates and develops them, they draw from the person and his moral values the indication of their purpose and the awareness of their limits.

It would on the one hand be illusory to claim that scientific research and its applications are morally neutral; on the other hand one cannot derive criteria for guidance from mere technical efficiency, from research's possible usefulness to some at the expense of others, or, worse still, from prevailing ideologies. Thus science and technology require, for their own intrinsic meaning, an unconditional respect for the fundamental criteria of the moral law: that is to say, they must be at the service of the human person, of his inalienable rights and his true and integral good according to the design and will of God.[7]

The rapid development of technological discoveries gives greater urgency to this need to respect the criteria just mentioned: science without conscience can only lead to man's ruin. "Our era needs such wisdom more than bygone ages if the discoveries made by man are to be further humanized. For the future of the world stands in peril unless wiser people are forthcoming."[8]

3. Anthropology and Procedures
in the Biomedical Field

What moral criteria must be applied in order to clarify the problems posed today in the field of biomedicine? The answer to this question presupposes a proper idea of the nature of the human person in his bodily dimension.

For it is only in keeping with his true nature that the human person can achieve self-realization as a "unified totality,"[9] and this nature is, at the same time, corporal and spiritual. By virtue of its substantial union with a spiritual soul, the human body cannot be considered as a mere complex of tissues, organs and functions, nor can it be evaluated in the same way as the body of animals; rather it is a constitutive part of the person who manifests and expresses himself through it.

The natural moral law expresses and lays down the purposes, rights and duties which are based upon the bodily and spiritual nature of the human person. Therefore this law cannot be thought of as simply a set of norms on the biological level; rather, it must be defined as the rational order whereby man is called by the Creator to direct and regulate his life and actions and, in particular, to make use of his own body.[10]

A first consequence can be deduced from these principles: an intervention on the human body affects not only the tissues, the organs and their functions, but also involves the person himself on different levels. It involves, therefore, perhaps in an implicit but nonetheless real way, a moral significance and responsibility. Pope John Paul II forcefully reaffirmed this to the World Medical Association when he said: "Each human person, in his absolutely unique singularity, is constituted not only by his spirit, but by his body as well. Thus, in the body and through the body, one touches the person himself in his concrete reality. To respect the dignity of man consequently amounts to safeguarding this identity of the man '*corpore et anima unus*,' as the Second Vatican Council says (*Gaudium et Spes*, 14, par. 1). It is on the basis of this anthropological vision that one is to find the fundamental criteria for decision making in the case of procedures which are not strictly therapeutic, as, for example, those aimed at the improvement of the human biological condition."[11]

Applied biology and medicine work together for the integral good of human life when they come to the aid of a person stricken by illness and infirmity and when they respect his or her dignity as a creature of God. No biologist or doctor can reasonably claim, by virtue of his scientific competence, to be able to decide on people's origin and destiny. This norm must be applied in a particular way in the field of sexuality and procreation, in which man and woman actualize the fundamental values of love and life.

God, who is love and life, has inscribed in man and woman the vocation to share in a special way in his mystery of personal communion and in his work as Creator and Father.[12] For this reason marriage possesses specific goods and values in its union and in procreation which cannot be likened to those existing in lower forms of life. Such values and meanings are of the personal order and determine from the moral point of view the meaning and limits of artificial interventions on procreation and on the origin of human life. These interventions are not to be rejected on the grounds that they are artificial. As such, they bear witness to the possibilities of the art of medicine. But they must be given a moral evaluation in reference to the dignity of the human person, who is called to realize his vocation from God to the gift of love and the gift of life.

4. Fundamental Criteria for a Moral Judgment

The fundamental values connected with the techniques of artificial human procreation are two: the life of the human being called into existence and the special nature of the transmission of human life in marriage. The moral judgment on such methods of artificial procreation must therefore be formulated in reference to these values.

Physical life, with which the course of human life in the world begins, certainly does not itself contain the whole of a person's value, nor does it represent the supreme good of man who is called to eternal life. However, it does constitute in a certain way the "fundamental" value of life, precisely because upon this physical life all the other values of the person are based and developed.[13] The inviolability of the innocent human being's right to life "from the moment of conception until death"[14] is a sign and requirement of the very inviolability of the person to whom the Creator has given the gift of life.

By comparison with the transmission of other forms of life in the universe, the transmission of human life has a special character of its own, which derives from the special nature of the human person. "The transmission of human life is entrusted by nature to a personal and conscious act and as such is subject to the all-holy laws of God: immutable and inviolable laws which must be recognized and observed. For this reason one cannot use means and follow methods which could be licit in the transmission of the life of plants and animals."[15]

Advances in technology have now made it possible to procreate apart from sexual relations through the meeting *in vitro* of the germ cells previously taken from the man and the woman. But what is technically possible is not for that very reason morally admissible. Rational reflection on the fundamental values of life and of human procreation is therefore indispensable for formulating a moral evaluation of such technological interventions on a human being from the first stages of his development.

5. Teachings of the Magisterium

On its part, the magisterium of the church offers to human reason in this field too the light of Revelation: the doctrine concerning man taught by the magisterium contains many elements which throw light on the problems being faced here.

From the moment of conception, the life of every human being is to be respected in an absolute way because man is the only creature on earth that God has "wished for himself"[16] and the spiritual soul of each man is "immediately created" by God;[17] his whole being bears the image of the Creator. Human life is sacred because from its beginning it involves "the creative action of God"[18] and it remains forever in a special relationship with the Creator, who is its sole end.[19] God alone is the Lord of life from its beginning until its end: no one can, in any circumstance, claim for himself the right to destroy directly an innocent human being.[20]

Human procreation requires on the part of the spouses responsible collaboration with the fruitful love of God;[21] the gift of human life must be actualized in marriage through the specific and exclusive acts of husband and wife, in accordance with the laws inscribed in their persons and in their union.[22]

I

Respect for Human Embryos

Careful reflection on this teaching of the magisterium and on the evidence of reason, as mentioned above, enables us to respond to the numerous moral problems posed by technical interventions upon the human being in the first phases of his life and upon the processes of his conception.

1. What respect is due to the human embryo, taking into account his nature and identity?

The human being must be respected—as a person—from the very first instant of his existence.

The implementation of procedures of artificial fertilization has made possible various interventions upon embryos and human fetuses. The aims pursued are of various kinds: diagnostic and therapeutic, scientific and commercial. From all of this, serious problems arise. Can one speak of a right to experimentation upon human embryos for the purpose of scientific research? What norms or laws should be worked out with regard to this matter? The response to these problems presupposes a detailed reflection on the nature and specific identity—the word "status" is used—of the human embryo itself.

At the Second Vatican Council, the church for her part presented once again to modern man her constant and certain doctrine, according to which, "Life once conceived, must be protected with the utmost care; abortion and infanticide are abominable crimes."[23] More recently, the *Charter of the Rights of the Family*, published by the Holy See, confirmed that "Human life must be absolutely respected and protected from the moment of conception."[24]

This Congregation is aware of the current debates concerning the beginning of human life, the individuality of the human being and the identity of the human person. The Congregation recalls the teachings found in the *Declaration on Procured Abortion*: "From the time that the ovum is fertilized, a new life is begun which is neither that of the father nor of the mother; it is rather the life of a new human being with his own growth. It would never be made human if it were not human already. To this perpetual evidence ... modern genetic science brings valuable confirmation. It has demonstrated that, from the first instant, the program is fixed as to what this living being will be: a man, this individual-man with his characteristic aspects already well determined. Right from fertilization is begun the adventure of a human life, and each of its great capacities requires time ... to find its place and to be in a position to act."[25] This teaching remains valid and is further confirmed, if confirmation were needed, by recent findings of human biological science which recognize that in the zygote* resulting from fertilization the biological identity of a new human individual is already constituted.

Certainly no experimental datum can be in itself sufficient to bring us to the recognition of a spiritual soul; nevertheless, the conclusions of science regarding the human embryo provide a valuable indication for discerning by the use of reason a personal presence at the moment of this first appearance of a human life: how could a human individual not be a human person? The magisterium has not expressly committed itself to an affirmation of a philosophical nature, but it constantly reaffirms the moral condemnation of any kind of procured abortion. This teaching has not been changed and is unchangeable.[26]

Thus the fruit of human generation, from the first moment of its existence, that is to say from the moment the zygote has formed, demands the unconditional respect that is morally due

---

* The zygote is the cell produced when the nuclei of the two gametes have fused.

to the human being in his bodily and spiritual totality. The human being is to be respected and treated as a person from the moment of conception; and therefore from that same moment his rights as a person must be recognized, among which in the first place is the inviolable right of every innocent human being to life.

This doctrinal reminder provides the fundamental criterion for the solution of the various problems posed by the development of the biomedical sciences in this field: since the embryo must be treated as a person, it must also be defended in its integrity, tended and cared for, to the extent possible, in the same way as any other human being as far as medical assistance is concerned.

2. IS PRENATAL DIAGNOSIS MORALLY LICIT?

If prenatal diagnosis respects the life and integrity of the embryo and the human fetus and is directed toward its safeguarding or healing as an individual, then the answer is affirmative.

For prenatal diagnosis makes it possible to know the condition of the embryo and of the fetus when still in the mother's womb. It permits, or makes it possible to anticipate earlier and more effectively, certain therapeutic, medical or surgical procedures.

Such diagnosis is permissible with the consent of the parents after they have been adequately informed, if the methods employed safeguard the life and integrity of the embryo and the mother, without subjecting them to disproportionate risks.[27] But this diagnosis is gravely opposed to the moral law when it is done with the thought of possibly inducing an abortion depending upon the results: a diagnosis which shows the existence of a malformation or a hereditary illness must not be the equivalent of a death sentence. Thus a woman would be committing a gravely illicit act if she were to request such a diagnosis with the deliberate intention of having an abortion should the results confirm the existence of a malformation or abnormality. The spouse or relatives or anyone else would similarly be acting in a manner contrary to the moral law if they were to counsel or impose such a diagnostic procedure on the expectant mother with the same intention of possibly proceeding to an abortion. So too the specialist would be guilty of illicit collaboration if, in conducting the diagnosis and in communicating its results, he were deliberately to contribute to establishing or favoring a link between prenatal diagnosis and abortion.

In conclusion, any directive or program of the civil and health authorities or of scientific organizations which in any way would favor a link between prenatal diagnosis and abortion, or which would go so far as directly to induce expectant mothers to submit to prenatal diagnosis planned for the purpose of eliminating fetuses which are affected by malformations or which are carriers of hereditary illness, is to be condemned as a violation of the unborn child's right to life and as an abuse of the prior rights and duties of the spouses.

3.   ARE THERAPEUTIC PROCEDURES CARRIED OUT ON THE HUMAN EMBRYO LICIT?

As with all medical interventions on patients, *one must uphold as licit procedures carried out on the human embryo which respect the life and integrity of the embryo and do not involve disproportionate risks for it but are directed toward its healing, the improvement of its condition of health, or its individual survival.*

Whatever the type of medical, surgical or other therapy, the free and informed consent of the parents is required, according to the deontological rules followed in the case of children. The application of this moral principle may call for delicate and particular precautions in the case of embryonic or fetal life.

The legitimacy and criteria of such procedures have been clearly stated by Pope John Paul II: "A strictly therapeutic intervention whose explicit objective is the healing of various maladies such as those stemming from chromosomal defects will, in principle, be considered desirable, provided it is directed to the true promotion of the personal well-being of the individual without doing harm to his integrity or worsening his conditions of life. Such an intervention would indeed fall within the logic of the Christian moral tradition."[28]

4. HOW IS ONE TO EVALUATE MORALLY RESEARCH AND EXPERI-
MENTATION* ON HUMAN EMBRYOS AND FETUSES?

Medical research must refrain from operations on live embryos,
unless there is a moral certainty of not causing harm to the life or
integrity of the unborn child and the mother, and on condition that
the parents have given their free and informed consent to the proce-
dure. It follows that all research, even when limited to the simple
observation of the embryo, would become illicit were it to involve
risk to the embryo's physical integrity or life by reason of the
methods used or the effects induced.

As regards experimentation, and presupposing the general
distinction between experimentation for purposes which are not
directly therapeutic and experimentation which is clearly therapeutic for the subject himself, in the case in point one must also
distinguish between experimentation carried out on embryos
which are still alive and experimentation carried out on embryos
which are dead. *If the embryos are living, whether viable or not,*
they must be respected just like any other human person; experi-
mentation on embryos which is not directly therapeutic is illicit.[29]

No objective, even though noble in itself, such as a foreseeable
advantage to science, to other human beings or to society, can in
any way justify experimentation on living human embryos or
fetuses, whether viable or not, either inside or outside the
mother's womb. The informed consent ordinarily required for
clinical experimentation on adults cannot be granted by the
parents, who may not freely dispose of the physical integrity or
life of the unborn child. Moreover, experimentation on embryos
and fetuses always involves risk, and indeed in most cases it

---

* Since the terms "research" and "experimentation" are often used equivalently and
ambiguously, it is deemed necessary to specify the exact meaning given them in this
document.

1) By *research* is meant *any* inductive-deductive process which aims at promoting the
systematic observation of a given phenomenon in the human field or at verifying a hypothesis arising from previous observations.

2) By *experimentation* is meant any research in which the human being (in various stages
of his existence: embryo, fetus, child or adult) represents the object through which or upon
which one intends to verify the effect, at present unknown or not sufficiently known, of
a given treatment (e.g. pharmacological, teratogenic, surgical, etc.).

involves the certain expectation of harm to their physical integrity
or even their death.

To use human embryos or fetuses as the object or instrument
of experimentation constitutes a crime against their dignity as
human beings having a right to the same respect that is due to
the child already born and to every human person.

The *Charter of the Rights of the Family* published by the Holy
See affirms: "Respect for the dignity of the human being excludes
all experimental manipulation or exploitation of the human
embryo."[30] The practice of keeping alive human embryos *in vivo*
or *in vitro* for experimental or commercial purposes is totally
opposed to human dignity.

In the case of experimentation that is clearly therapeutic,
namely, when it is a matter of experimental forms of therapy used
for the benefit of the embryo itself in a final attempt to save its
life, and in the absence of other reliable forms of therapy,
recourse to drugs or procedures not yet fully tested can be licit.[31]

*The corpses of human embryos and fetuses, whether they have
been deliberately aborted or not, must be respected just as the remains
of other human beings.* In particular, they cannot be subjected to
mutilation or to autopsies if their death has not yet been verified
and without the consent of the parents or of the mother. Furthermore, the moral requirements must be safeguarded that there be
no complicity in deliberate abortion and that the risk of scandal
be avoided. Also, in the case of dead fetuses, as for the corpses
of adult persons, all commercial trafficking must be considered
illicit and should be prohibited.

5. HOW IS ONE TO EVALUATE MORALLY THE USE FOR RESEARCH
    PURPOSES OF EMBRYOS OBTAINED BY FERTILIZATION 'IN
    VITRO'?

Human embryos obtained *in vitro* are human beings and
subjects with rights: their dignity and right to life must be
respected from the first moment of their existence. *It is immoral
to produce human embryos destined to be exploited as disposable
"biological material."*

In the usual practice of *in vitro* fertilization, not all of the
embryos are transferred to the woman's body; some are destroyed.

Just as the church condemns induced abortion, so she also forbids acts against the life of these human beings. *It is a duty to condemn the particular gravity of the voluntary destruction of human embryos obtained 'in vitro' for the sole purpose of research, either by means of artificial insemination or by means of "twin fission."* By acting in this way the researcher usurps the place of God; and, even though he may be unaware of this, he sets himself up as the master of the destiny of others inasmuch as he arbitrarily chooses whom he will allow to live and whom he will send to death and kills defenseless human beings.

Methods of observation or experimentation which damage or impose grave and disproportionate risks upon embryos obtained *in vitro* are morally illicit for the same reasons. Every human being is to be respected for himself, and cannot be reduced in worth to a pure and simple instrument for the advantage of others. *It is therefore not in conformity with the moral law deliberately to expose to death human embryos obtained 'in vitro'.* In consequence of the fact that they have been produced *in vitro*, those embryos which are not transferred into the body of the mother and are called "spare" are exposed to an absurd fate, with no possibility of their being offered safe means of survival which can be licitly pursued.

6. WHAT JUDGMENT SHOULD BE MADE ON OTHER PROCEDURES OF MANIPULATING EMBRYOS CONNECTED WITH THE "TECHNIQUES OF HUMAN REPRODUCTION"?

Techniques of fertilization *in vitro* can open the way to other forms of biological and genetic manipulation of human embryos, such as attempts or plans for fertilization between human and animal gametes and the gestation of human embryos in the uterus of animals, or the hypothesis or project of constructing artificial uteruses for the human embryo. *These procedures are contrary to the human dignity proper to the embryo, and at the same time they are contrary to the right of every person to be conceived and to be born within marriage and from marriage.*[32] Also, attempts or hypotheses for obtaining a human being without any connection with sexuality through "twin fission," cloning or parthenogenesis are to

*be considered contrary to the moral law, since they are in opposition
to the dignity both of human procreation and of the conjugal union.*

The freezing of embryos, even when carried out in order to
preserve the life of an embryo—cryopreservation—*constitutes an
offense against the respect due to human beings* by exposing them
to grave risks of death or harm to their physical integrity and
depriving them, at least temporarily, of maternal shelter and
gestation, thus placing them in a situation in which further
offenses and manipulation are possible.

*Certain attempts to influence chromosomic or genetic inheritance
are not therapeutic but are aimed at producing human beings
selected according to sex or other predetermined qualities. These
manipulations are contrary to the personal dignity of the human
being and his or her integrity and identity.* Therefore in no way
can they be justified on the grounds of possible beneficial consequences for future humanity.[33] Every person must be respected
for himself: in this consists the dignity and right of every human
being from his or her beginning.

II

INTERVENTIONS UPON HUMAN PROCREATION

By "artificial procreation" or "artificial fertilization" are understood here the different technical procedures directed toward obtaining a human conception in a manner other than the sexual union of man and woman. This Instruction deals with fertilization of an ovum in a test tube (*in vitro* fertilization) and artificial insemination through transfer into the woman's genital tracts of previously collected sperm.

A preliminary point for the moral evaluation of such technical procedures is constituted by the consideration of the circumstances and consequences which those procedures involve in relation to the respect due the human embryo. Development of the practice of *in vitro* fertilization has required innumerable fertilizations and destructions of human embryos. Even today, the usual practice presupposes a hyperovulation on the part of the woman; a number of ova are withdrawn, fertilized and then cultivated *in vitro* for some days. Usually not all are transferred into the genital tracts of the woman; some embryos, generally called "spare," are destroyed or frozen. On occasion, some of the implanted embryos are sacrificed for various eugenic, economic or psychological reasons. Such deliberate destruction of human beings or their utilization for different purposes to the detriment of their integrity and life is contrary to the doctrine on procured abortion already recalled.

The connection between *in vitro* fertilization and the voluntary destruction of human embryos occurs too often. This is significant:

through these procedures, with apparently contrary purposes, life and death are subjected to the decision of man, who thus sets himself up as the giver of life and death by decree. This dynamic of violence and domination may remain unnoticed by those very individuals who, in wishing to utilize this procedure, become subject to it themselves. The facts recorded and the cold logic which links them must be taken into consideration for a moral judgment of IVF and ET (*in vitro* fertilization and embryo transfer): the abortion mentality which has made this procedure possible thus leads, whether one wants it or not, to man's domination over the life and death of his fellow human beings and can lead to a system of radical eugenics.

Nevertheless, such abuses do not exempt one from a further and thorough ethical study of the techniques of artificial procreation considered in themselves, abstracting as far as possible from the destruction of embryos produced *in vitro*.

The present Instruction will therefore take into consideration in the first place the problems posed by heterologous artificial fertilization (II, 1-3),* and subsequently those linked with homologous artificial fertilization (II, 4-6).**

Before formulating an ethical judgment on each of these procedures, the principles and values which determine the moral evaluation of each of them will be considered.

---

* By the term *heterologous artificial fertilization or procreation,* the Instruction means techniques used to obtain a human conception artificially by the use of gametes coming from at least one donor other than the spouses who are joined in marriage. Such techniques can be of two types:

a) *Heterologous IVF and ET:* the technique used to obtain a human conception through the meeting *in vitro* of gametes taken from at least one donor other than the two spouses joined in marriage.

b) *Heterologous artificial insemination:* the technique used to obtain a human conception through the transfer into the genital tracts of the woman of the sperm previously collected from a donor other than the husband.

** By *artificial homologous fertilization or procreation,* the Instruction means the technique used to obtain a human conception using the gametes of the two spouses joined in marriage. Homologous artificial fertilization can be carried out by two different methods:

a) *Homologous IVF and ET:* the technique used to obtain a human conception through the meeting *in vitro* of the gametes of the spouses joined in marriage.

b) *Homologous artificial insemination:* the technique used to obtain a human conception through the transfer into the genital tracts of a married woman of the sperm previously collected from her husband.

A
HETEROLOGOUS ARTIFICIAL FERTILIZATION

1. WHY MUST HUMAN PROCREATION TAKE PLACE IN MARRIAGE?

Every human being is always to be accepted as a gift and blessing of God. However, from the moral point of view a truly responsible procreation vis-à-vis the unborn child must be the fruit of marriage.

For human procreation has specific characteristics by virtue of the personal dignity of the parents and of the children: the procreation of a new person, whereby the man and woman collaborate with the power of the Creator, must be the fruit and sign of the mutual self-giving of the spouses, of their love and their fidelity.[34] *The fidelity of the spouses in the unity of marriage involves reciprocal respect of their right to become a father and a mother only through each other.*

The child has the right to be conceived, carried in the womb, brought into the world and brought up within marriage: it is through the secure and recognized relationship to his own parents that the child can discover his own identity and achieve his own proper human development.

The parents find in their child a confirmation and completion of their reciprocal self-giving: the child is the living image of their love, the permanent sign of their conjugal union, the living and indissoluble concrete expression of their paternity and maternity.[35]

By reason of the vocation and social responsibilities of the person, the good of the children and of the parents contributes to the good of civil society; the vitality and stability of society require that children come into the world within a family and that the family be firmly based on marriage.

The tradition of the church and anthropological reflection recognize in marriage and in its indissoluble unity the only setting worthy of truly responsible procreation.

2. DOES HETEROLOGOUS ARTIFICIAL FERTILIZATION CONFORM TO THE DIGNITY OF THE COUPLE AND TO THE TRUTH OF MARRIAGE?

Through IVF and ET and heterologous artificial insemination, human conception is achieved through the fusion of gametes of at least one donor other than the spouses who are united in marriage. *Heterologous artificial fertilization is contrary to the unity of marriage, to the dignity of the spouses, to the vocation proper to parents, and to the child's right to be conceived and brought into the world in marriage and from marriage.*[36]

Respect for the unity of marriage and for conjugal fidelity demands that the child be conceived in marriage; the bond existing between husband and wife accords the spouses, in an objective and inalienable manner, the exclusive right to become father and mother solely through each other.[37] Recourse to the gametes of a third person, in order to have sperm or ovum available, constitutes a violation of the reciprocal commitment of the spouses and a grave lack in regard to that essential property of marriage which is its unity.

Heterologous artificial fertilization violates the rights of the child; it deprives him of his filial relationship with his parental origins and can hinder the maturing of his personal identity. Furthermore, it offends the common vocation of the spouses who are called to fatherhood and motherhood: it objectively deprives conjugal fruitfulness of its unity and integrity; it brings about and manifests a rupture between genetic parenthood, gestational parenthood and responsibility for upbringing. Such damage to the personal relationships within the family has repercussions on civil society: what threatens the unity and stability of the family is a source of dissension, disorder and injustice in the whole of social life.

These reasons lead to a negative moral judgment concerning heterologous artificial fertilization: consequently, fertilization of a married woman with the sperm of a donor different from her husband and fertilization with the husband's sperm of an ovum not coming from his wife are morally illicit. Furthermore, the artificial fertilization of a woman who is unmarried or a widow, whoever the donor may be, cannot be morally justified.

The desire to have a child and the love between spouses who long to obviate a sterility which cannot be overcome in any other way constitute understandable motivations; but subjectively good intentions do not render heterologous artificial fertilization conformable to the objective and inalienable properties of marriage or respectful of the rights of the child and of the spouses.

3. IS "SURROGATE"* MOTHERHOOD MORALLY LICIT?

No, for the same reasons which lead one to reject heterologous artificial fertilization: for it is contrary to the unity of marriage and to the dignity of the procreation of the human person.

Surrogate motherhood represents an objective failure to meet the obligations of maternal love, conjugal fidelity and responsible motherhood; it offends the dignity and right of the child to be conceived, carried in the womb, brought into the world and brought up by his own parents; it sets up, to the detriment of families, a division between the physical, psychological and moral elements which constitute those families.

---

* By "surrogate mother" the Instruction means:

a) the woman who carries in pregnancy an embryo implanted in her uterus and who is genetically a stranger to the embryo because it has been obtained through the union of the gametes of "donors." She carries the pregnancy with a pledge to surrender the baby once it is born to the party who commissioned or made the agreement for the pregnancy.

b) the woman who carries in pregnancy an embryo to whose procreation she has contributed the donation of her own ovum, fertilized through insemination with the sperm of a man other than her husband. She carries the pregnancy with a pledge to surrender the child once it is born to the party who commissioned or made the agreement for the pregnancy.

B
HOMOLOGOUS ARTIFICIAL FERTILIZATION

Since heterologous artificial fertilization has been declared unacceptable, the question arises of how to evaluate morally the process of homologous artificial fertilization: IVF and ET and artificial insemination between husband and wife. First a question of principle must be clarified.

4. WHAT CONNECTION IS REQUIRED FROM THE MORAL POINT OF VIEW BETWEEN PROCREATION AND THE CONJUGAL ACT?

a) The church's teaching on marriage and human procreation affirms the "inseparable connection, willed by God and unable to be broken by man on his own initiative, between the two meanings of the conjugal act: the unitive meaning and the procreative meaning. Indeed, by its intimate structure, the conjugal act, while most closely uniting husband and wife, capacitates them for the generation of new lives, according to laws inscribed in the very being of man and of woman."[38] This principle, which is based upon the nature of marriage and the intimate connection of the goods of marriage, has well-known consequences on the level of responsible fatherhood and motherhood. "By safeguarding both these essential aspects, the unitive and the procreative, the conjugal act preserves in its fullness the sense of true mutual love and its ordination toward man's exalted vocation to parenthood."[39]

The same doctrine concerning the link between the meanings of the conjugal act and between the goods of marriage throws light on the moral problem of homologous artificial fertilization, since "it is never permitted to separate these different aspects to such a degree as positively to exclude either the procreative intention or the conjugal relation."[40]

Contraception deliberately deprives the conjugal act of its openness to procreation and in this way brings about a voluntary dissociation of the ends of marriage. Homologous artificial fertilization, in seeking a procreation which is not the fruit of a specific act of conjugal union, objectively effects an analogous separation between the goods and the meanings of marriage.

Thus, *fertilization is licitly sought when it is the result of a "conjugal act which is per se suitable for the generation of children to which marriage is ordered by its nature and by which the spouses become one flesh."*[41] But from the moral point of view, procreation is deprived of its proper perfection when it is not desired as the fruit of the conjugal act, that is to say, of the specific act of the spouses' union.

b) The moral value of the intimate link between the goods of marriage and between the meanings of the conjugal act is based upon the unity of the human being, a unity involving body and spiritual soul.[42] Spouses mutually express their personal love in the "language of the body," which clearly involves both "spousal meanings" and parental ones.[43] The conjugal act by which the couple mutually express their self-gift at the same time expresses openness to the gift of life. It is an act that is inseparably corporal and spiritual. It is in their bodies and through their bodies that the spouses consummate their marriage and are able to become father and mother. In order to respect the language of their bodies and their natural generosity, the conjugal union must take place with respect for its openness to procreation; and the procreation of a person must be the fruit and result of married love. The origin of the human being thus follows from a procreation that is "linked to the union, not only biological but also spiritual, of the parents, made one by the bond of marriage."[44] Fertilization achieved outside the bodies of the couple remains by this very fact deprived of the meanings and values which are expressed in the language of the body and in the union of human persons.

c) Only respect for the link between the meanings of the conjugal act and respect for the unity of the human being make possible procreation in conformity with the dignity of the person. In his unique and irrepeatable origin, the child must be respected and recognized as equal in personal dignity to those who give him life. The human person must be accepted in his parents' act of union and love; the generation of a child must therefore be the fruit of that mutual giving[45] which is realized in the conjugal act wherein the spouses cooperate as servants and not as masters in the work of the Creator who is Love.[46]

In reality, the origin of a human person is the result of an act of giving. The one conceived must be the fruit of his parents' love. He cannot be desired or conceived as the product of an intervention of medical or biological techniques; that would be equivalent to reducing him to an object of scientific technology. No one may subject the coming of a child into the world to conditions of technical efficiency which are to be evaluated according to standards of control and dominion.

The moral relevance of the link between the meanings of the conjugal act and between the goods of marriage, as well as the unity of the human being and the dignity of his origin, demand that the procreation of a human person be brought about as the fruit of the conjugal act specific to the love between spouses. The link between procreation and the conjugal act is thus shown to be of great importance on the anthropological and moral planes, and it throws light on the positions of the magisterium with regard to homologous artificial fertilization.

5. IS HOMOLOGOUS 'IN VITRO' FERTILIZATION MORALLY LICIT?

The answer to this question is strictly dependent on the principles just mentioned. Certainly one cannot ignore the legitimate aspirations of sterile couples. For some, recourse to homologous IVF and ET appears to be the only way of fulfilling their sincere desire for a child. The question is asked whether the totality of conjugal life in such situations is not sufficient to ensure the dignity proper to human procreation. It is acknowledged that IVF and ET certainly cannot supply for the absence of sexual relations[47] and cannot be preferred to the specific acts of conjugal union, given the risks involved for the child and the difficulties of the procedure. But it is asked whether, when there is no other way of overcoming the sterility which is a source of suffering, homologous *in vitro* fertilization may not constitute an aid, if not a form of therapy, whereby its moral licitness could be admitted.

The desire for a child—or at the very least an openness to the transmission of life—is a necessary prerequisite from the moral point of view for responsible human procreation. But this good intention is not sufficient for making a positive moral evaluation of *in vitro* fertilization between spouses. The process of IVF and ET must be judged in itself and cannot borrow its definitive moral quality from the totality of conjugal life of which it becomes part nor from the conjugal acts which may precede or follow it.[48]

It has already been recalled that, in the circumstances in which it is regularly practiced, IVF and ET involves the destruction of human beings, which is something contrary to the doctrine on the illicitness of abortion previously mentioned.[49] But even in a situation in which every precaution were taken to avoid the death of human embryos, homologous IVF and ET dissociates from the conjugal act the actions which are directed to human fertilization. For this reason the very nature of homologous IVF and ET also must be taken into account, even abstracting from the link with procured abortion.

Homologous IVF and ET is brought about outside the bodies of the couple through actions of third parties whose competence and technical activity determine the success of the procedure. Such fertilization entrusts the life and identity of the embryo to the power of doctors and biologists, and establishes the domination of technology over the origin and destiny of the human person. Such a relationship of domination is in itself contrary to the dignity and equality that must be common to parents and children.

Conception *in vitro* is the result of the technical action which presides over fertilization. *Such fertilization is neither in fact achieved nor positively willed as the expression and fruit of a specific act of the conjugal union. In homologous IVF and ET, therefore, even if it is considered in the context of 'de facto' existing sexual relations, the generation of the human person is objectively deprived of its proper perfection: namely, that of being the result and fruit of a conjugal act* in which the spouses can become "cooperators with God for giving life to a new person."[50]

These reasons enable us to understand why the act of conjugal love is considered in the teaching of the church as the only setting worthy of human procreation. For the same reasons the so-called "simple case," i.e. a homologous IVF and ET procedure that is free of any compromise with the abortive practice of destroying embryos and with masturbation, remains a technique which is morally illicit because it deprives human procreation of the dignity which is proper and connatural to it.

Certainly, homologous IVF and ET fertilization is not marked by all that ethical negativity found in extraconjugal procreation; the family and marriage continue to constitute the setting for the birth and upbringing of the children. Nevertheless, in conformity with the traditional doctrine relating to the goods of marriage and the dignity of the person, *the church remains opposed from the moral point of view to homologous 'in vitro' fertilization. Such fertilization is in itself illicit and in opposition to the dignity of procreation and of the conjugal union, even when everything is done to avoid the death of the human embryo.*

Although the manner in which human conception is achieved with IVF and ET cannot be approved, every child which comes into the world must in any case be accepted as a living gift of the divine Goodness and must be brought up with love.

6. HOW IS HOMOLOGOUS ARTIFICIAL INSEMINATION TO BE EVALUATED FROM THE MORAL POINT OF VIEW?

Homologous artificial insemination within marriage cannot be admitted except for those cases in which the technical means is not a substitute for the conjugal act but serves to facilitate and to help so that the act attains its natural purpose.

The teaching of the magisterium on this point has already been stated.[51] This teaching is not just an expression of particular historical circumstances but is based on the church's doctrine concerning the connection between the conjugal union and procreation and on a consideration of the personal nature of the conjugal act and of human procreation. "In its natural structure, the conjugal act is a personal action, a simultaneous and immediate cooperation on the part of the husband and wife, which by the very nature of the agents and the proper nature of the act is the expression of the mutual gift which, according to the words of Scripture, brings about union 'in one flesh'."[52] Thus moral conscience "does not necessarily proscribe the use of certain artificial means destined solely either to the facilitating of the natural act or to ensuring that the natural act normally performed achieves its proper end."[53] If the technical means facilitates the conjugal act or helps it to reach its natural objectives, it can be morally acceptable. If, on the other hand, the procedure were to replace the conjugal act, it is morally illicit.

Artificial insemination as a substitute for the conjugal act is prohibited by reason of the voluntarily achieved dissociation of the two meanings of the conjugal act. Masturbation, through which the sperm is normally obtained, is another sign of this dissociation: even when it is done for the purpose of procreation, the act remains deprived of its unitive meaning: "It lacks the sexual relationship called for by the moral order, namely the relationship which realizes 'the full sense of mutual self-giving and human procreation in the context of true love'."[54]

7. WHAT MORAL CRITERION CAN BE PROPOSED WITH REGARD TO MEDICAL INTERVENTION IN HUMAN PROCREATION?

The medical act must be evaluated not only with reference to its technical dimension but also and above all in relation to its goal, which is the good of persons and their bodily and psychological health. The moral criteria for medical intervention in procreation are deduced from the dignity of human persons, of their sexuality and of their origin.

Medicine which seeks to be ordered to the integral good of the person must respect the specifically human values of sexuality.[55] *The doctor is at the service of persons and of human procreation. He does not have the authority to dispose of them or to decide their fate.* A medical intervention respects the dignity of persons when it seeks to assist the conjugal act either in order to facilitate its performance or in order to enable it to achieve its objective once it has been normally performed."[56]

On the other hand, it sometimes happens that a medical procedure technologically replaces the conjugal act in order to obtain a procreation which is neither its result nor its fruit. In this case the medical act is not, as it should be, at the service of conjugal union but rather appropriates to itself the procreative function and thus contradicts the dignity and inalienable rights of the spouses and of the child to be born.

The humanization of medicine, which is insisted upon today by everyone, requires respect for the integral dignity of the human person first of all in the act and at the moment in which the spouses transmit life to a new person. It is only logical, therefore, to address an urgent appeal to Catholic doctors and scientists that they bear exemplary witness to the respect due to the human embryo and to the dignity of procreation. The medical and nursing staff of Catholic hospitals and clinics are in a special way urged to do justice to the moral obligations which they have also frequently assumed as part of their contract. Those who are in charge of Catholic hospitals and clinics and who are often religious will take special care to safeguard and promote a diligent observance of the moral norms recalled in the present Instruction.

8. THE SUFFERING CAUSED BY INFERTILITY IN MARRIAGE

The suffering of spouses who cannot have children or who are afraid of bringing a handicapped child into the world is a suffering that everyone must understand and properly evaluate.

On the part of the spouses, the desire for a child is natural: it expresses the vocation to fatherhood and motherhood inscribed in conjugal love. This desire can be even stronger if the couple is affected by sterility which appears incurable. Nevertheless, marriage does not confer upon the spouses the right to have a child, but only the right to perform those natural acts which are *per se* ordered to procreation.[57]

A true and proper right to a child would be contrary to the child's dignity and nature. The child is not an object to which one has a right, nor can he be considered as an object of ownership: rather, a child is a gift, "the supreme gift"[58] and the most gratuitous gift of marriage, and is a living testimony of the mutual giving of his parents. For this reason, the child has the right, as already mentioned, to be the fruit of the specific act of the conjugal love of his parents; and he also has the right to be respected as a person from the moment of his conception.

Nevertheless, whatever its cause or prognosis, sterility is certainly a difficult trial. The community of believers is called to shed light upon and support the suffering of those who are unable to fulfill their legitimate aspiration to motherhood and fatherhood. Spouses who find themselves in this sad situation are called to find in it an opportunity for sharing in a particular way in the Lord's cross, the source of spiritual fruitfulness. Sterile couples must not forget that "even when procreation is not possible, conjugal life does not for this reason lose its value. Physical sterility in fact can be for spouses the occasion for other important services to the life of the human person, for example, adoption, various forms of educational work, and assistance to other families and to poor or handicapped children."[59]

Many researchers are engaged in the fight against sterility. While fully safeguarding the dignity of human procreation, some have achieved results which previously seemed unattainable. Scientists therefore are to be encouraged to continue their research with the aim of preventing the causes of sterility and of being able to remedy them so that sterile couples will be able to procreate in full respect for their own personal dignity and that of the child to be born.

III

MORAL AND CIVIL LAW

The Values and Moral Obligations that Civil Legislation Must Respect and Sanction in this Matter

The inviolable right to life of every innocent human individual and the rights of the family and of the institution of marriage constitute fundamental moral values, because they concern the natural condition and integral vocation of the human person; at the same time they are constitutive elements of civil society and its order.

For this reason the new technological possibilities which have opened up in the field of biomedicine require the intervention of the political authorities and of the legislator, since an uncontrolled application of such techniques could lead to unforeseeable and damaging consequences for civil society. Recourse to the conscience of each individual and to the self-regulation of researchers cannot be sufficient for ensuring respect for personal rights and public order. If the legislator responsible for the common good were not watchful, he could be deprived of his prerogatives by researchers claiming to govern humanity in the name of the biological discoveries and alleged "improvement" processes which they would draw from those discoveries. "Eugenics" and forms of discrimination between human beings could become legitimized: this would constitute an act of violence and a serious offense to the equality, dignity and fundamental rights of the human person.

The intervention of the public authority must be inspired by the rational principles which regulate the relationships between civil law and moral law. The task of the civil law is to ensure the common good of people through the recognition and defense of fundamental rights and through the promotion of peace and public morality.[60] In no sphere of life can the civil law take the place of conscience or dictate norms concerning things which are outside its competence. It must sometimes tolerate, for the sake of public order, things which it cannot forbid without a greater evil resulting. However, the inalienable rights of the person must be recognized and respected by civil society and the political authority. These human rights depend neither on single individuals nor on parents; nor do they represent a concession made by society and the state: they pertain to human nature and are inherent in the person by virtue of the creative act from which the person took his or her origin.

Among such fundamental rights one should mention in this regard: *a)* every human being's right to life and physical integrity from the moment of conception until death; *b)* the rights of the family and of marriage as an institution and, in this area, the child's right to be conceived, brought into the world and brought up by his parents. It is necessary here to give some further consideration to each of these two themes.

In various states certain laws have authorized the direct suppression of innocents: the moment a positive law deprives a category of human beings of the protection which civil legislation must accord them, the state is denying the equality of all before the law. When the state does not place its power at the service of the rights of each citizen, and in particular of the more vulnerable, the very foundations of a state based on law are undermined. The political authority consequently cannot give approval to the calling of human beings into existence through procedures which would expose them to those very grave risks noted previously. The possible recognition by positive law and the political authorities of techniques of artificial transmission of life and the experimentation connected with it would widen the breach already opened by the legalization of abortion.

As a consequence of the respect and protection which must be ensured for the unborn child from the moment of his conception, the law must provide appropriate penal sanctions for every deliberate violation of the child's rights. The law cannot tolerate—indeed it must expressly forbid—that human beings, even at the embryonic state, should be treated as objects of experimentation, be mutilated or destroyed with the excuse that they are superfluous or incapable of developing normally.

The political authority is bound to guarantee to the institution of the family, upon which society is based, the juridical protection to which it has a right. From the very fact that it is at the service of people, the political authority must also be at the service of the family. Civil law cannot grant approval to techniques of artificial procreation which, for the benefit of third parties (doctors, biologists, economic or governmental powers), take away what is a right inherent in the relationship between spouses; and therefore civil law cannot legalize the donation of gametes between persons who are not legitimately united in marriage.

Legislation must also prohibit, by virtue of the support which is due to the family, embryo banks, *post mortem* insemination and "surrogate motherhood."

It is part of the duty of the public authority to ensure that the civil law is regulated according to the fundamental norms of the moral law in matters concerning human rights, human life and the institution of the family. Politicians must commit themselves, through their interventions on public opinion, to securing in society the widest possible consensus on such essential points and to consolidating this consensus wherever it risks being weakened or is in danger of collapse.

In many countries, the legalization of abortion and juridical tolerance of unmarried couples make it more difficult to secure respect for the fundamental rights recalled by this Instruction. It is to be hoped that states will not become responsible for aggravating these socially damaging situations of injustice. It is rather to be hoped that nations and states will realize all the cultural, ideological and political implications connected with the techniques of artificial procreation and will find the wisdom and courage necessary for issuing laws which are more just and more respectful of human life and the institution of the family.

The civil legislation of many states confers an undue legitimation upon certain practices in the eyes of many today; it is seen to be incapable of guaranteeing that morality which is in conformity with the natural exigencies of the human person and with the "unwritten laws" etched by the Creator upon the human heart. All men of good will must commit themselves, particularly within their professional field and in the exercise of their civil rights, to ensuring the reform of morally unacceptable civil laws and the correction of illicit practices. In addition, "conscientious objection" vis-à-vis such laws must be supported and recognized. A movement of passive resistance to the legitimation of practices contrary to human life and dignity is beginning to make an ever sharper impression upon the moral conscience of many, especially among specialists in the biomedical sciences.

CONCLUSION

The spread of technologies of intervention in the processes of human procreation raises very serious moral problems in relation to the respect due to the human being from the moment of conception, to the dignity of the person, of his or her sexuality, and of the transmission of life.

With this Instruction the Congregation for the Doctrine of the Faith, in fulfilling its responsibility to promote and defend the church's teaching in so serious a matter, addresses a new and heartfelt invitation to all those who, by reason of their role and their commitment, can exercise a positive influence and ensure that, in the family and in society, due respect is accorded to life and love. It addresses this invitation to those responsible for the formation of consciences and of public opinion, to scientists and medical professionals, to jurists and politicians. It hopes that all will understand the incompatibility between recognition of the dignity of the human person and contempt for life and love, between faith in the living God and the claim to decide arbitrarily the origin and fate of a human being.

In particular, the Congregation for the Doctrine of the Faith addresses an invitation with confidence and encouragement to theologians, and above all to moralists, that they study more deeply and make ever more accessible to the faithful the contents of the teaching of the church's magisterium in the light of a valid anthropology in the matter of sexuality and marriage and in the context of the necessary interdisciplinary approach. Thus they will make it possible to understand ever more clearly the reasons for and the validity of this teaching. By defending man against the excesses of his own power, the church of God reminds him of the reasons for his true nobility; only in this way can the possibility of living and loving with that dignity and liberty which derive from respect for the truth be ensured for the men and women of tomorrow. The precise indications offered in the present Instruction therefore are not meant to halt the effort of reflection but rather to give it a renewed impulse in unrenounceable fidelity to the teaching of the church.

In the light of the truth about the gift of human life and in the light of the moral principles which flow from that truth, everyone is invited to act in the area of responsibility proper to each and, like the good Samaritan, to recognize as a neighbor even the littlest among the children of men (cf. Lk 10:29-37). Here Christ's words find a new and particular echo: "What you do to one of the least of my brethren, you do unto me" (Mt 25:40).

During an audience granted to the undersigned Prefect after the plenary session of the Congregation for the Doctrine of the Faith, the Supreme Pontiff, John Paul II, approved this Instruction and ordered it to be published.

Given at Rome, from the Congregation for the Doctrine of the Faith, February 22, 1987, the Feast of the Chair of St. Peter, the Apostle.

Joseph Card. Ratzinger
Prefect

✟ Alberto Bovone
Titular Archbishop of Caesarea in Numidia
Secretary

Notes

1. Pope John Paul II, Discourse to participants in the 81st Congress of the Italian Society of Internal Medicine and the 82nd Congress of the Italian Society of General Surgery, 27 October 1980, *AAS* 72 (1980):1126.

2. Pope John Paul VI, Discourse to the General Assembly of the United Nations Organization, 4 October 1965, *AAS* 57 (1965):878; Encyclical *Populorum Progressio*, 13, *AAS* 59 (1967): 263.

3. Pope Paul VI, Homily during the Mass closing the Holy Year, 25 December 1975, *AAS* 68 (1976):145; Pope John Paul II, Encyclical *Dives in Misericordia*, 30, *AAS* 72 (1980):1224.

4. Pope John Paul II, Discourse to participants in the 35th General Assembly of the World Medical Association, 29 October 1983, *AAS* 76 (1984):390.

5. Cf. Declaration *Dignitatis Humanae* 2.

6. Pastoral Constitution *Gaudium et Spes*, 22; Pope John Paul II, Encyclical *Redemptor Hominis*, 8, *AAS* 71 (1979):270-72.

7. Cf. Pastoral Constitution *Gaudium et Spes*, 35.

8. Pastoral Constitution *Gaudium et Spes*, 15; cf. also Pope Paul VI, Encyclical *Populorum Progressio*, 20, *AAS* 59 (1967):267; Pope John Paul II, Encyclical *Redemptor Hominis*, 15, *AAS* 71 (1979):286-89; Apostolic Exhortation *Familiaris Consortio*, 8, *AAS* 74 (1982):89.

9. Pope John Paul II, Apostolic Exhortation *Familiaris Consortio*, 11, *AAS* 74 (1982):92.

10. Cf. Pope Paul VI, Encyclical *Humanae Vitae*, 10, *AAS* 60 (1968):487-88.

11. Pope John Paul II, Discourse to members of the 35th General Assembly of the World Medical Association, 29 October 1983, *AAS* 76 (1984):393.

12. Cf. Pope John Paul II, Apostolic Exhortation *Familiaris Consortio*, 11, *AAS* 74 (1982):91-92; cf. also Pastoral Constitution *Gaudium et Spes*, 50.

13. Sacred Congregation for the Doctrine of the Faith, *Declaration on Procured Abortion*, 9, *AAS* 66 (1974):736-37.

14. Pope John Paul II, Discourse to participants in the 35th General Assembly of the World Medical Association, 29 October 1983, *AAS* 76 (1984):390.

15. Pope John XXIII, Encyclical *Mater et Magistra*, III, *AAS* 53 (1961):447.

16. Pastoral Constitution *Gaudium et Spes*, 24.

17. Cf. Pope Pius XII, Encyclical *Humani Generis*, *AAS* 42 (1950):575; Pope Paul VI, *Professio Fidei*, *AAS* 60 (1968):436.

18. Pope John XXIII, Encyclical *Mater et Magistra*, III, *AAS* 53 (1961):447; cf. Pope John Paul II, Discourse to priests participating in a seminar on "Responsible Procreation," 17 September 1983, *Insegnamenti di Giovanni Paolo II*, VI, 2 (1983):562: "At the origin of each human person there is a creative act of God: no man comes into existence by chance; he is always the result of the creative love of God."

19. Cf. Pastoral Constitution *Gaudium et Spes*, 24.

20. Cf. Pope Pius XII, *Discourse to the Saint Luke Medical-Biological Union*, 12 November 1944: *Discorsi e Radiomessaggi VI* (1944-1945):191-92.

21. Cf. Pastoral Constitution *Gaudium et Spes*, 50.

22. Cf. Pastoral Constitution *Gaudium et Spes*, 51: "When it is a question of harmonizing married love with the responsible transmission of life, the moral character of one's behavior does not depend only on the good intention and the evaluation of the motives: objective criteria must be used, criteria drawn from the nature of the human person and human acts, criteria which respect the total meaning of mutual self-giving and human procreation in the context of true love."

23. Pastoral Constitution *Gaudium et Spes*, 51.

24. Holy See, *Charter of the Rights of the Family*, 4: *L'Osservatore Romano*, 25 November 1983.

25. Sacred Congregation for the Doctrine of the Faith, *Declaration on Procured Abortion*, 12-13, *AAS* 66 (1974):738.

26. Cf. Pope Paul VI, Discourse to participants in the 23rd National Congress of Italian Catholic Jurists, 9 December 1972, *AAS* 64 (1972):777.

27. The obligation to avoid disproportionate risks involves an authentic respect for human beings and the uprightness of therapeutic intentions. It implies that the doctor "above all... must carefully evaluate the possible negative consequences which the necessary use of a particular exploratory technique may have upon the unborn child and avoid recourse to diagnostic procedures which do not offer sufficient guarantees of their honest purpose and substantial harmlessness. And if, as often happens in human choices, a degree of risk must be undertaken, he will take care to assure that it is justified by a truly urgent need for the diagnosis and by the importance of the results that can be achieved by it for the benefit of the unborn himself" (Pope John Paul II, 3 December 1982: *Insegnamenti di Giovanni Paolo II*, V, 3 [1982]: 1512). This clarification concerning "proportionate risk" is also to be kept in mind in the following sections of the present Instruction, whenever this term appears.

28. Pope John Paul II, Discourse to participants in the 35th General Assembly of the World Medical Association, 29 October 1983, *AAS* 76 (1984):392.

29. Cf. Pope John Paul II, Address to a meeting of the Pontifical Academy of Sciences, 23 October 1982, *AAS* 75 (1983):37: "I condemn, in the most explicit and formal way, experimental manipulations of the human embryo, since the human being, from conception to death, cannot be exploited for any purpose whatsoever."

30. Holy See, *Charter of the Rights of the Family*, 4b: *L'Osservatore Romano*, 25 November 1983.

31. Cf. Pope John Paul II, Address to participants in the Convention of the Pro-Life Movement, 3 December 1982: *Insegnamenti di Giovanni Paolo II*, V, 3 (1982):1511: "Any form of experimentation on the fetus that may damage its integrity or worsen its condition is unacceptable, except in the case of a final effort to save it from death." Sacred Congregation for the Doctrine of the Faith, *Declaration on Euthanasia*, 4, *AAS* 72 (1980):550: "In the absence of other sufficient remedies, it is permitted, with the patient's consent, to have recourse to the means provided by the most advanced medical techniques, even if these means are still at the experimental stage and are not without a certain risk."

32. No one, before coming into existence, can claim a subjective right to begin to exist; nevertheless, it is legitimate to affirm the right of the child to have a fully human origin through conception in conformity with the personal nature of the human being. Life is a gift that must be bestowed in a manner worthy both of the subject receiving it and of the subjects transmitting it. This statement is to be borne in mind also for what will be explained concerning artificial human procreation.

33. Cf. Pope John Paul II, Discourse to participants in the 35th General Assembly of the World Medical Association, 29 October 1983, *AAS* 76 (1984):391.

34. Cf. Pastoral Constitution *Gaudium et Spes*, 50.

35. Cf. Pope John Paul II, Apostolic Exhortation *Familiaris Consortio*, 14, *AAS* 74 (1982):96.

36. Cf. Pope Pius XII, Discourse to participants in the 4th International Congress of Catholic Doctors, 29 September 1949: *AAS* 41 (1949):559. According to the plan of the Creator, "A man leaves his father and his mother and cleaves to his wife, and they become one flesh" (Gn 2:24). The unity of marriage, bound to the order of creation, is a truth accessible to natural reason. The church's tradition and magisterium frequently make reference to the book of Genesis, both directly and through the passages of the New

Testament that refer to it, Mt 19:46; Eph 5:31. Cf. Athenagoras, *Legatio pro christianis*, 33: PG 6, 965-967; St. Chrysostom, *In Matthaeum homiliae*, LXII, 19, 1: PG 58, 597; St. Leo the Great, *Epist. ad Rusticum*, 4: PL 54, 1204; Innocent III, *Epist. Gaudemus in Domino*: DS 778; Council of Lyons II, IV Session: DS 860; Council of Trent, XXIV Session: DS 1798, 1802; Pope Leo XIII, Encyclical *Arcanum Divinae Sapientiae, ASS* 12 (1879/80):388-91; Pope Pius XI, Encyclical *Casti Connubii, AAS* 22 (1930):546-47; Second Vatican Council, *Gaudium et Spes*, 48; Pope John Paul II, Apostolic Exhortation *Familiaris Consortio*, 19, *AAS* 74 (1982):101-02; *Code of Canon Law*, Can. 1056.

37. Cf. Pope Pius XII, Discourse to participants in the 4th International Congress of Catholic Doctors, 29 September 1949, *AAS* 41 (1949):560; Discourse to participants in the Congress of the Italian Catholic Union of Midwives, 29 October 1951, *AAS* 43 (1951):850; *Code of Canon Law*, Can. 1134.

38. Pope Paul VI, Encyclical Letter *Humanae Vitae*, 12, *AAS* 60 (1968):488-89.

39. Ibid., 489.

40. Pope Pius XII, Discourse to participants in the Second Naples World Congress on Fertility and Human Sterility, 19 May 1956, *AAS* 48 (1956):470.

41. *Code of Canon Law*, Can. 1061. According to this canon, the conjugal act is that by which the marriage is consummated if the couple "have performed (it) between themselves in a human manner."

42. Cf. Pastoral Constitution *Gaudium et Spes*, 14.

43. Cf. Pope John Paul II, General Audience on 16 January 1980: *Insegnamenti di Giovanni Paolo II*, III, I (1980):148-52.

44. Pope John Paul II, Discourse to participants in the 35th General Assembly of the World Medical Association, 29 October 1983, *AAS* 76 (1984):393.

45. Cf. Pastoral Constitution *Gaudium et Spes*, 51.

46. Cf. Pastoral Constitution *Gaudium et Spes*, 50.

47. Cf. Pope Pius XII, Discourse to participants in the 4th International Congress of Catholic Doctors, 29 September 1949, *AAS* 41 (1949):560: "it would be erroneous... to think that the possibility of resorting to this means [artificial fertilization] might render valid a marriage between persons unable to contract it because of the *impedimentum impotentiae*."

48. A similar question was dealt with by Pope Paul VI, Encyclical *Humanae Vitae*, 14, *AAS* 60 (1968):490-91.

49. Cf. above: I, 1 ff.

50. Pope Paul II, Apostolic Exhortation *Familiaris Consortio*, 14, *AAS* 74 (1982):96.

51. *Response of the Holy Office*, 17 March 1897: DS 3323; Pope Pius XII, Discourse to participants in the 4th International Congress of Catholic Doctors, 29 September 1949, *AAS* 41 (1949):560; Discourse to the Italian Catholic Union of Midwives, 29 October 1951, *AAS* 43 (1951):850; Discourse to participants in the Second Naples World Congress on Fertility and Human Sterility, 19 May 1956, *AAS* 48 (1956):471-73; Discourse to those taking part in the 7th International Congress of the International Society of Hematology, 12 September 1958, *AAS* 50 (1958):733; Pope John XXIII, Encyclical *Mater et Magistra*, III, *AAS* 53 (1961):447.

52. Pope Pius XII, Discourse to the Italian Catholic Union of Midwives, 29 October 1951, *AAS* 43 (1951):850.

53. Pope Pius XII, Discourse to participants in the 4th International Congress of Catholic Doctors, 29 September 1949, *AAS* 41 (1949):560.

54. Sacred Congregation for the Doctrine of the Faith, *Declaration on Certain Questions Concerning Sexual Ethics*, 9, *AAS* 68 (1976):86, which quotes the Pastoral Constitution *Gaudium et Spes*, 51. Cf. *Decree of the Holy Office*, 2 August 1929, *AAS* 21 (1929):490; Pope Pius XII, Discourse to those taking part in the 26th Congress of the Italian Society of Urology, 8 October 1953, *AAS* 45 (1953):678.

55. Cf. Pope John XXIII, Encyclical *Mater et Magistra*, III, *AAS* 53 (1961):447.

56. Cf. Pope Pius XII, Discourse to participants in the 4th International Congress of Catholic Doctors, 29 September 1949, *AAS* 41 (1949):560.

57. Cf. Pope Pius XII, Discourse to participants in the Second Naples World Congress on Fertility and Human Sterility, 19 May 1956, *AAS* 48 (1956):471-73.

58. Pastoral Constitution *Gaudium et Spes*, 50.

59. Pope John Paul II, Apostolic Exhortation *Familiaris Consortio*, 14, *AAS* 74 (1982):97.

60. Cf. Declaration *Dignitatis Humanae*, 7.

II

CLINICAL AND
TECHNICAL ASPECTS

JOHN COLLINS HARVEY, M.D., Ph.D.

An Introduction to the Biological and Medical Aspects of In Vitro Fertilization

The document *Instruction on Respect for Human Life in Its Origin and On the Dignity of Procreation* was issued by the Sacred Congregation for the Doctrine of the Faith in March of 1987. It is popularly known as *Donum Vitae*. It is authoritative magisterial teaching and as such is an important guideline to all people of God. The document is opposed from the moral point of view to homologous in vitro fertilization, that is, in vitro fertilization within marriage. Prior to the issuance of the document many Catholic obstetricians and health care facilities had carried on programs of homologous in vitro fertilization. These were considered as medical benefits to childless couples whose infertility could be treated by these highly sophisticated and recently developed techniques which when successful brought great joy to an infertile couple. This result was indeed considered by the physician as a "good" which was part of his/her duty in his/her role of healer. The joy that resulted from this therapeutic triumph perhaps was best expressed by Pope John Paul I when he sent a telegram welcoming Louise Brown, the first baby born as a result of in vitro fertilization, into this world.

Donum Vitae's opposition to homologous in vitro fertilization is not based on a rejection of technical manipulation, for in the Introduction there is the statement: "These interventions are not to be rejected on the grounds that they are artificial. As such they bear witness to the possibilities of the art of medicine." The Instruction says: "they must be given a moral evaluation in reference to the dignity of the human person who is called to realize his vocation to God, to the gift of love, and the gift of life."

We know that the dignity of the human person is part of the divine plan or eternal law in the mind of God, our Creator and Redeemer. This is well understood in the Thomistic view of natural law now leavened by a twentieth century anthropological approach fully consistent with the teaching of the Second Vatican Council (*Gaudium et Spes*, 14, para. 1). As part of the eternal law there is natural law or "right reason," which is reason directing us to our ultimate end in accordance with our nature. This is the participation of the rational creature in the eternal law.

Truth may be found, Thomas asserted, on the basis of human reasoning reflecting on human nature in the light of faith. The human person understands himself/herself as a moral being. The physician necessarily understands that medical ethical conduct is moral conduct. Since medical problems are human problems, they often present moral problems. Medical problems do not have a moral solution because God in whom we believe has ordained things in a particular fashion. Medical ethics are not revealed! Rather, questions of what medical conduct and actions correspond to humanity have to be solved on the basis of the self-understanding of the human person.

The human person must explore and discover. The God of faith is not irrelevant in our search to find solutions. The God who created us and redeemed us wills our search to be a search that gives solutions which truly correspond to our humanity created freely as a loving gift of God, a totally self-sufficient, self-fulfilled God. This faith from which moral action (or for physicians, medical ethics) proceeds is not an assertion of the truth of certain propositions but an act deep in the person of entrusting himself/herself to God, who reveals and imparts himself to us. God seeks our salvation and has given us redemption. His concern for us is that we be open to others and to all that is good. Jesus' way in the world was doing good, helping others, and healing.

Thus, the physician's attempt to develop himself/herself in relation to medical ethics is an attempt that derives from faith. But faith and theological anthropology cannot replace human philosophical reflection. It is true, also, that in seeking a Catholic medical ethics on the basis of faith, all Catholic physicians may not arrive at the same conclusions. Medical ethical principles are not objects of faith but must be discovered "in the light of the Gospel." But faith does have a maieutic function. Faith enables reason to ask the correct questions.

There are certain fundamental and believed truths relative to a Catholic medical ethics. These are:

1. God has created human beings.
2. We are made in His image.
3. All human beings share in His love.
4. In the life, death, and resurrection of Jesus all human beings have been transformed into new creatures.
5. The ultimate significance and dignity of all human beings consists in developing this new life in his love.
6. The Spirit is given to us to guide and inspire us on our pilgrimage to our everlasting home, heaven.
7. Each individual must be open to others in this new life in Christ's love which shapes itself in justice, understanding, and forbearance.

When truths are to be made concrete, human reflection begins. In the past it was thought that such reflections were made not only in "the light of the Gospel" but under the guidance of the Holy Spirit. As such, they were thought to be free from error. Today we have different judgments with regard to moral solutions in the Christian tradition. Catholic moral theologians have given different answers to different questions at different periods. Authoritative magisterial teaching has reflected such theological input.

The teaching of medical ethics has seen us standing in ultimate relationship to the doctrine of the faith of the church. The church, then, as the guardian of faith, intervenes in an official way in moral theology, that is, in medical ethics. But the doctrine of the faith of the church does not contain concrete answers to moral questions. The church has no special knowledge in certain areas such as human sexuality, embryology, genetic composition and the like.

Knowledge about these matters comes from human reflection and is presupposed in moral affirmation about human behavior. Noninfallible authoritative magisterial teaching includes statements which are not found in the treasury of the church's faith. The church's magisterium rightly insists that one must adhere to such teaching in forming conscience. Biologists, physicians, and theologians feel bound for instruction and praxis by the statements.

Catholic tradition has always emphasized mediation. God who reveals himself to us does so through a mediator. In the first covenant God revealed himself to us in the salvation history of his chosen people, Israel; in the law given to Moses on Mt. Sinai; and through the words of the prophets. In the second covenant, God has revealed himself in the created man, Jesus, our brother (conceived in the womb of our Blessed Mother, the virgin Mother, by the Holy Spirit without means of human sexual intercourse); and in the same person is the Christ, the uncreated logos of God, co-eternal with the Father and Spirit whose enfleshment, suffering, death, resurrection, and return to the Father has redeemed us and assured us salvation. God continues to reveal himself through the intermediary of the kingdom which Jesus established on earth, the church, and through its sacraments. The will of God is thus made known through and in human nature.

The theologian attempts to incorporate proven scientific results into his framework, comprehension and interpretation. There can be no contradiction between faith and scientific knowledge. There can be contradiction, however, between theological theory and scientific theory. One can think correctly about God only as long as one thinks correctly about his creation which is good (Gn 1:31).

The findings of the natural sciences do give theologians things to think about. They change the thinker's concept of self indirectly and immediately. The intellectual challenge for the moral theologian is that normative knowledge might establish a paradigm appropriate at one time but no longer. Change in the paradigm is the consequence of empirical research. It is also a consequence of the interface and interference with philosophical and theological interpretative schemes previously held.

The marvelous advances in molecular biology and medical practice have changed our concepts of biological life in the same fashion that the brilliant advances in astronomy have changed our concepts of the cosmos. The role of the physician is to apply these biological and medical advances to the clinical situation, to bring cure for disease, and, if such be not feasible, comfort, care and relief from suffering, both physical and mental, when possible. This is entirely consistent with the dignity of the human being and the role of the physician as mediator. Just as Jesus healed in his earthy ministry, so the physician must heal in his vocational calling.

Medical science has developed a technique to overcome a certain type of sterility in married couples specifically when the oviducts of the wife are absent or are totally obstructed by a disease process. Eggs can be harvested from the ovaries of the wife under certain conditions and may be fertilized in vitro by the sperm of the husband obtained by masturbation. This process is called in vitro fertilization or IVF. The fertilized eggs may then be transferred back to the wife's womb and proceed to develop as a normal pregnancy or pregnancies. This process is known as embryo transfer or ET. The Instruction indicates that such fertilization is in itself illicit and in opposition to the dignity of procreation and of the conjugal union even when everything is done to avoid the death of the human embryos. The argument offered in the Instruction is that this procedure separates the procreative aspect from the unitive aspect embodied in the act of human marital intercourse. The Instruction in its conclusion invites scientists, theologians, and philosophers to continue to explore and develop techniques which are morally consistent with the gift of love and the gift of life. The Instruction says in the third paragraph of the conclusion: "In particular, the Congregation for the Doctrine of the Faith addresses an invitation with confidence and encouragement to theologians, and above all moralists, that they study more deeply and make ever more accessible to the faithful the contents of the teaching of the church's magisterium in the light of a valid anthropology in the matter of sexuality and marriage and in the context of the necessary interdisciplinary approach."

Responding to this invitation, the Georgetown University Medical School and the Kennedy Institute of Ethics at the University jointly convened a conference of knowledgeable physicians, clerics, theologians, and philosophers to review the theological thought contained in the document. In the spirit of humility and obedience, the philosophical and theological arguments presented in the document were extensively studied.

To serve as a background for this exploration and for the education of the theologians and the philosophers in the scientific aspects of this medical treatment, the first part of the conference was a thorough in-depth presentation by two distinguished obstetricians-endocrinologists who are very knowledgeable in the field of reproductive technologies and who are internationally known as experts in the field of in vitro fertilization.

The first paper of the conference was a description of the medical aspects of in vitro fertilization given by Dr. Marian Damewood, Assistant Professor of Gynecology and Obstetrics at the Johns Hopkins University. Dr. Damewood is director of the in vitro fertilization program at the Johns Hopkins Hospital in Baltimore, Maryland. She is one of the outstanding obstetricians in North America working in this field. In addition, she is internationally recognized for her work and writings on the subject of IVF. In her presentation she described in a very clear and uncomplicated way the medical techniques used in this treatment for infertility. Her explanation for in vitro fertilization step by step provided a clear exposition of this medical treatment. It made explicit to the nonphysicians and nonbiologists present at the conference all of the aspects of this treatment—the medical rationale for its use, the technical aspects, the outcomes of the treatment, and those factors which affect outcomes. She educated the theologians and philosophers at the conference so that they understood the exact methodologies employed in this medical procedure.

The second presentation was given by Dr. Johannes Huber, Fasharzt and University Dozent in Gynecology and Obstetrics at the University of Vienna. Dr. Huber is also the director of the in vitro fertilization program at the famous Allgemeines Krankenhaus in Vienna. He, like Dr. Damewood, is recognized internationally as a leader in the field of IVF. His publications on the subject are numerous and are recognized for their clarity and reasoned thought. In addition to his medical degree earned at the University of Vienna, Dr. Huber also earned a doctorate in theology at the same institution. Dr. Huber, a prodigious worker, carried out fully his duties at the Allgemeines Krankenhaus and in the Medical School of the University of Vienna during his predoctoral and postdoctoral medical studies from 1973 through 1983, yet during the same period of time served as personal secretary to the Cardinal-Archbishop of Vienna, Cardinal Franz Koenig!

In his presentation Dr. Huber explained in a clear and explicit way some theologically informed modifications to the medical techniques routinely employed in in vitro fertilization which were described by Dr. Damewood. Dr. Huber felt that these modified processes might, from the theological perspective, bring IVF into conformity with the theological dicta of the Instruction and thus make IVF a licit treatment. Very importantly, Dr. Huber also described the latest observations on the development of the human embryo, observations which have been made possible by the technique of IVF. He described in great detail and emphasized the very important new knowledge regarding the lag in time between the insemination of a human oocyte with human sperm and the actual fertilization, i.e. the molecular process whereby the genetic material contained in the sperm of the father merges, within the oocyte (since the sperm has already penetrated the wall of the egg), with the genetic material of the mother to form the new and distinct genetic combination "becoming a human being." The timing of this process of syngamy, Dr. Huber explained, may offer a new paradigm for philosophers and theologians to utilize when they consider the morality of the simultaneous or separated aspects of procreation and union in the act of marital intercourse. These new biological observations, Dr. Huber offered, give us a deeper normative knowledge concerning the process of human fertilization. This knowledge will, in turn, contribute to an enrichment of theological and philosophical perspectives on the subject. This will be part of those medical, theological, and philosophical considerations made in full filial and obedient affection for the church, which have been requested by *Donum Vitae*.

These two papers serve then as the introduction to this volume. They clarify the biological and medical aspects of the process known as in vitro fertilization. They serve to bring the most recent scientific knowledge to theologians and philosophers for their consideration in deliberations concerning the morality of homologous in vitro fertilization.

MARIAN D. DAMEWOOD, M.D.

Current Technology of In Vitro Fertilization and Alternate Forms of Reproduction

I. Introduction

It has now been nine years since the birth of Louise Brown, the first baby conceived through the in vitro fertilization process. Since that time the technique of in vitro fertilization and embryo transfer has offered hope for married couples previously thought to be unable to conceive. However, since this first successful pregnancy, basic in vitro fertilization has expanded into areas of reproduction involving additional new technologies. These new technologies have stimulated much discussion about their efficacy and their ethical ramifications. The purpose of this paper is to describe the current technology of in vitro fertilization and its associated alternate forms of reproduction which are available at centers throughout the world. In order to consider these subjects, it is important to define the terms now generally accepted by scientists working in the field. Table 1 gives such important definitions.

II. Patient Candidates for In Vitro Fertilization

Married couples who enter into in vitro fertilization programs are typically at the "end stage" of infertility therapy. The major indication, therefore, for in vitro fertilization is failure of conventional surgical or medical therapy for infertility. The original indication for in vitro fertilization was loss of both fallopian tubes as a result of ectopic pregnancies. Since the late 1970s this

Table 1. Definitions.

IVF-ET: In vitro fertilization and embryo transfer. Procedure involving removal of eggs from the female. Laboratory fertilization with sperm from the male and transfer of embryos back to the female uterus.

Egg/Oocyte: An oocyte or ovum in the unfertilized state.

Pre-embryo: Product of the gametic union, from fertilization to the appearance of the embryonic axis. The pre-embryonic state is considered to last until fourteen days after fertilization. This definition is not intended to imply a moral evaluation of the pre-embryo.[1,2,3]

Gift: Gamete intrafallopian transfer. A procedure by which eggs are obtained from the female, sperm from the male, and both gametes placed back into the fallopian tube where fertilization occurs.[4]

Follicle: A structure which is approximately 2 cm in size arising on the ovary which contains an egg or oocyte.

Follicular Stimulation/Induction of Ovulation: Procedure by which fertility drugs are administered to stimulate the development of multiple follicles and multiple eggs. The normal female produces only one egg per month. With in vitro fertilization or GIFT procedures, five to seven eggs or more may be stimulated.[5,6,7]

---

indication has expanded to women with failed reconstructive tubal surgery or pelvic adhesions with extensive tubal damage. Other infertility problems in the female, such as endometriosis refractory to hormonal and surgical therapy, have also been successfully treated with IVF. Additional indications have included severe cervical factor, oligospermia, immunologic factors and unexplained infertility. Multiple causes of infertility such as a combination of tubal disease and oligospermia may also be included for therapy in an IVF program. The causes of infertility in the marital couples enrolled in the Johns Hopkins Hospital IVF Program are summarized in Table 2.

Table 2. Indications for IVF-ET, Johns Hopkins Hospital program.

1. Tubal occlusion/failed reconstructive tubal surgery
2. Endometriosis unresponsive to medical/surgical therapy
3. Absent fallopian tubes
4. Unexplained infertility
5. Oligospermia
6. Immunologic factors
7. Cervical factor

The assessment of couples for in vitro fertilization includes not only medical indication but also consideration of the couples' marital relationship.[8] Those couples requesting in vitro fertilization at the Johns Hopkins Hospital are required to obtain a psychologic evaluation prior to initiation of the IVF procedures.[9] The purpose of this evaluation is to assess the psychological strengths and weaknesses of the marriage relative to the expected stress of IVF procedures as well as its result, which will be either a successful pregnancy or failure to achieve pregnancy. It should be noted that in the Johns Hopkins Hospital's in vitro fertilization program only married couples are considered for admission. When alternate forms of reproduction are considered, still, in the majority of cases, only married couples are admitted; however, sources of sperm or oocytes other than the marital partners may be utilized.

III. Technology of Basic In Vitro Fertilization

Step 1. Ovulation Induction. Most in vitro fertilization programs use some type of medication to augment the number of fertilizable oocytes or eggs developed. Although the first successful in vitro pregnancy did result from the use of one egg obtained from a spontaneous natural cycle, the natural cycle has several disadvantages, including the difficulty in timing the release and subsequent retrieval of only one oocyte. The recruitment of multiple follicles and thus multiple eggs has allowed for the major advantage of making available many oocytes for fertilization and making possible the development of multiple embryos for transfer. This procedure facilitates an increase in pregnancy rates. The objective of this type of stimulation is to recruit a number of follicles between day 3 and 5 of a normal twenty-eight-day menstrual cycle. This time is noted as the "FSH stimulation window." Drugs used for this type of ovulation induction include clomiphen citrate, human menopausal gonadotropin (HMG), a combination of these agents or pure follicle stimulating hormone (pure FSH). In the Johns Hopkins Hospital's program, human menopausal gonadotropin and pure FSH are used in dosage of one to four ampules per day beginning on day 3 of the cycle through day 12. With this regimen, four to six oocytes per cycle have been obtained. With this regimen pregnancy rates at world centers range from 20 to 26%. Using the natural cycle is less expensive and requires less of the wife's time in the hospital. In the stimulated cycle, ovulation is regulated and the medication may cause the release of more than one egg, all of which can then be captured at the time of needle aspiration. The disadvantages of the stimulated cycle, however, are its increased expense and its requirement for longer stays in the hospital or clinic.

Step 2. Oocyte or Egg Retrieval. The eggs thus stimulated in the previous step can be harvested by laparoscopy or ultrasound guided needle puncture of the ovary.[10] Laparoscopic technology involves passing an operating laparoscope through the patient's umbilicus, making a second puncture in the patient's abdomen through which a grasping instrument is passed to hold down the ovary. An aspiration needle is then passed through the laparoscope and is inserted onto the ovarian follicle. Suction is then applied to the needle by a syringe. (See Figures 1 and 2.) This suction creates a negative pressure in the needle. The eggs are sucked into the needle in their follicular fluid and thus are captured. This technique has achieved an egg recovery rate of 89 to 94%.

A newer technique in use for IVF oocyte retrieval includes follicular puncture by a needle guided by sonograph.[11] In this

Figure 1. Laparoscopic technique to harvest oocytes.

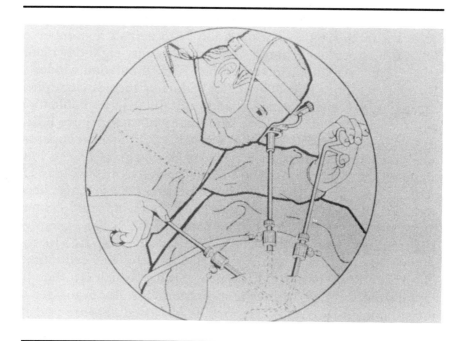

system, the ultrasound machine will calculate a line from the puncture site to the ovary through which a needle can be passed to aspirate the oocytes. The puncture may be achieved through the patient's bladder or more recently by a method utilizing a probe in the vaginal fornix.[12,13] Use of ultrasonic guidance has achieved precise localization of follicles on the ovarian surface, the exact location of the oocytes within the follicle, and has permitted oocyte retrieval rates of 80 to 90% per follicle.[14,15] The advantages of this ultrasonic guidance are several. It eliminates both general anesthesia and abdominal surgery for the patient.

Figure 2. Technique of aspirating oocytes from ovarian follicle.

1. Body of uterus; 2. & 3. Fallopian tubes; 4. Fimbria; 5. Ovary;
6. Ripe ovarian follicle

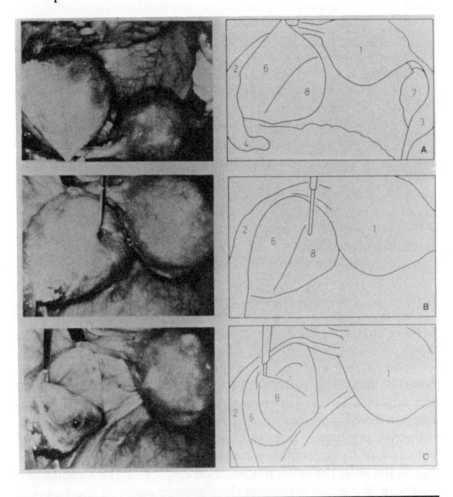

Step 3. Oocyte Fertilization and Development. Oocytes collected at operative or ultrasonic retrieval are evaluated immediately in the laboratory under the microscope for maturity and morphology. Mature eggs are fertilized in a sterile petri dish four to six hours after retrieval, with approximately 50,000 motile sperm from the husband's sperm specimen obtained by masturbation and provided on the day of the wife's surgery. These inseminated eggs are evaluated daily for evidence of fertilization. Cleaving (or dividing) embryos at the two- to four-cell stage are transferred to the patient forty-eight to seventy-two hours after retrieval. The embryo transfer is performed using a small catheter placed through the cervix into the uterus through which the embryos are transferred by syringe injection. Pregnancy success rates per embryo transfer have ranged from 10 to 30% depending on the number of embryos transferred. With one embryo transfer, the pregnancy rate is approximately 10%, but with three to four cleaving embryos, success rates are currently 25% per cycle. It should be emphasized that presently in the Johns Hopkins Hospital's program all healthy eggs and embryos removed from a woman are transferred back to her uterus.

There is a discrepancy in the timing of the maturation of the embryo fertilized in vitro when compared to the embryo fertilized in vivo. It takes approximately 150 hours to achieve the blastomere state when fertilized in vitro as compared to 105 hours to achieve this state for the embryo fertilized in vivo. (See Figure 3.)

The current expectation of pregnancy is in the range of 25%, based on treatment cycles with transfers. This pregnancy rate and the miscarriage rate differ somewhat but not widely from those rates observed in normal (in vivo) reproduction. The factors which influence pregnancy rates per treatment cycle are the following: the cause of the infertility, the mobility of sperm at screening, the age of the wife, the induction method employed, the number and maturity of oocytes collected, the cleavage status of the embryos developed, the number of embryos transferred into the uterus, the difficulties encountered in transfer, and the age of the embryos at transfer.

Figure 3. Discrepancy in embryo maturation after in vivo and in vitro fertilization.

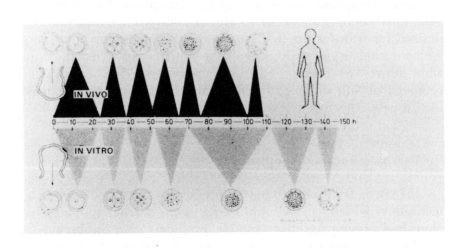

IV. New Techniques—Embryo Cryopreservation

In many programs the problem of disposition of a large number of cleaving embryos has arisen when drugs have been employed as noted above to stimulate egg production. There are many options for utilization of these large numbers of eggs or embryos, including:

1. transferring all embryos to the wife's uterus (presently required in the Johns Hopkins program protocol);
2. limiting the number of the eggs recovered or inseminated;
3. preserving eggs or embryos for future transfer.

This latter action has allowed the wife opportunity to have embryo transfer at a later natural cycle. Successful pregnancies have been reported in 8 to 10% of patients who have had embryos frozen and later transferred.[16] Factors affecting the success rate of the procedure include the number of embryos frozen, their developmental stage at freezing, and "normality" of the embryos when examined under the microscope just prior to transfer. Cryopreservation of eggs or embryos is also utilized in situations where numbers of oocytes or embryos in excess of those desired for transfer for IVF are obtained. Cryopreservation may be a solution to the serious problem which arises when the wife who desires to preserve fertility must have diseased ovaries removed or will undergo radiation or chemotherapy for cancer in the pelvic region or even elsewhere.[17]

V. Alternate Forms of Reproduction

In vitro fertilization has stimulated the development of techniques which can be employed to treat marital couples who have had previously uncorrectable problems such as absence of sperm in the husband, or absence of eggs or even absence of the uterus in the wife. These alternate avenues of reproduction are listed in Table 3.

Table 3. Alternate avenues of reproduction.

1. Use of donor eggs
2. Use of donor sperm
3. Donation of pre-embryos
4. Surrogate mothers
5. Surrogate uterus

In vitro fertilization has also opened many investigative opportunities to observe egg and sperm interaction and to study the early phases of human development. However, these technologies are associated with unprecedented ethical dilemmas. These technologies impose responsibilities upon the gynecologist-reproductive endocrinologist which were not present a decade ago and for which there is little guidance. Specifically, these research areas include:

- observation of early events in fertilization, i.e. sperm egg fusion and interaction;
- experimental evaluation of the pre-embryo, including blastomere biopsy (cell removal);
- genetic manipulation of the pre-embryo by chromosomal analysis and/or gene insertion.

While these technological and research areas have the potential for major contributions to unknown areas of human reproduction, they remain extremely controversial in medical, legal, and ethical arenas.

The GIFT Procedure. The GIFT (or gamete intrafallopian transfer) procedure has been thought by some investigators to be a more physiologic approach than in vitro fertilization.[18] In this situation, patients who have normal fallopian tubes may have their eggs and their husband's sperm placed back into the fallopian tube in a simple operative procedure. Thus, GIFT involves placement of both gametes, i.e. sperm and eggs, into the fallopian tube. The procedure is very similar in the first two steps to the techniques employed in in vitro fertilization, viz. induction of multiple follicular development and removal of eggs through the laparoscope. In the GIFT procedure, however, after the husband's sperm is obtained, both the harvested eggs and the sperm are drawn up into a teflon catheter and the mixture of eggs and sperm is then placed back into the wife's fallopian tube through the laparoscope. Should there be blockage in the fallopian tube, the placement of the mixture of eggs and sperm is distal to the blockage. Fertilization in this situation occurs not in the laboratory petri dish, as with in vitro fertilization, but in the patient's fallopian tube, which is the usual site of fertilization in vivo. (See Figure 4.)

The first GIFT procedure reported was successful. It produced twin girls. Utilizing this technique, the pregnancy rate at present is 35% per attempt. The GIFT technique may be a more physiologic approach than IVF inasmuch as the ampullary region of the

Figure 4. GIFT procedure.

---

a. Ovulation induction
b. Harvesting of oocytes by laparoscopic technique
c. Catheter collection of eggs and sperm separated by air bubble partition.
d. Insertion of eggs and sperm into the fallopian tube.

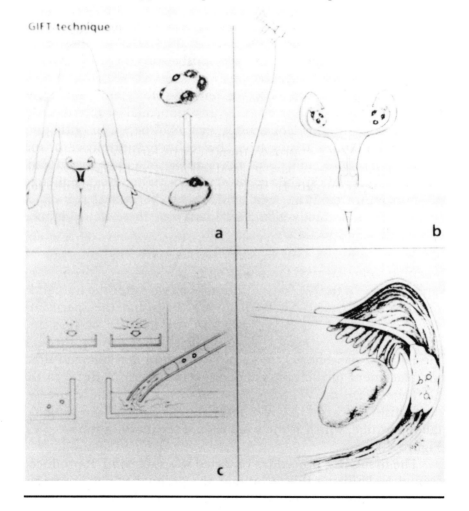

GIFT technique

fallopian tube is the normal site of fertilization in the human. Patients with unexplained infertility or mild endometriosis may be candidates for this procedure because, in these cases, failure of spermatozoa to reach the tube may be the cause of infertility. The GIFT procedure is now widely used when the fallopian anatomy is appropriate.

VI. Conclusion

In vitro fertilization and its associated technology is of significance in reproduction because it does offer an alternative to what was thought to be previously intractable infertility. However, this new technology, as well as its associated alternate forms of reproduction, have given rise to many important concerns. One such concern is with "noncoital" reproduction. Another concern involves actions that may be taken with pre-embryos. Questions arising from this technology are new, for the extracorporeal pre-embryo has never before had to be considered. Our technological capabilities present us with the great challenge of enunciating medical, legal and, above all, ethical principles which will guide analysis and evaluation of these new methods of human reproduction.[19]

Notes

1. Ethics Committee of the American Fertility Society, "Ethical Considerations on the New Reproduction Technologies," *Fertility and Sterility* 46:1 (1986).

2. The Instruction *Donum Vitae* does attribute identical moral status to the pre-embryo, zygote, embryo and fetus. See note in the Foreword to the Instruction.

3. According to the Ethics Committee of the American Fertility Society, a pre-embryo is a product of gametic union from fertilization to the appearance of the embryonic axis. The pre-embryotic stage is considered to last until fourteen days after fertilization. This definition is not intended to imply a moral evaluation of the pre-embryo. In this paper the use of "embryo" does imply moral status. The term "egg" is used in the generic sense to mean either an oocyte or ovum in the unfertilized state. See notes 1 and 2 above.

4. R.H. Asch, J.P. Balmaceda, L.R. Ellsworth, P.C. Wong, "Gamete Intrafallopian Transfer (GIFT): A New Treatment for Infertility," *International Journal of Fertility* 30:41 (1985).

5. R.E. Barnardus, G.S. Jones, A.A. Acosta, J.E. Garcia, H.C. Lui, D.L. Jones, Z. Rosenwaks, "The Significance of the Ratio in Follicle-stimulating Hormone and Luteinizing Hormone in Induction of Multiple Follicular Growth," *Fertility and Sterility* 43:373 (1985).

6. M.D. Damewood, E.E. Wallach, "IVF Update," *Postgraduate Obstetrics and Gynecology* 6:1 (1986).

7. M.D. Damewood, E.E. Wallach, "Latest Techniques Improve IVF Success Rates," *Contemporary OB/GYN Technology* (1987).

8. M.D. Damewood, "In Vitro Fertilization and Psychosexual Aspects," *Journal of Clinical Practice in Sexuality* (forthcoming).

9. P.J. Fagan, C.W. Schmidt, Jr., J.A. Rock, M.D. Damewood, E. Halle, T.N. Wise, "Sexual Functioning and Psychologic Evaluation of In Vitro Fertilization Couples," *Fertility and Sterility* 46:668 (1986).

10. W. Feichtinger, P. Kemeter, "Laparoscopic or Ultrasonically Guided Follicle Aspiration for In Vitro Fertilization," *Journal of In Vitro Fertilization and Embryo Transfer* 1:244 (1984).

11. P. Dellenbach, I. Nisand, L. Moreau, B. Feger, C. Plumere, P. Gerlinger, "Transvaginal Sonographically Controlled Follicle Puncture for Oocyte Retrieval," *Fertility and Sterility* 44:656 (1985).

12. S. Lenz, J.G. Lauritsen, "Ultrasonically Guided Percutaneous Aspiration of Human Follicles under Local Anesthesia: A New Method of Collecting Oocytes for In Vitro Fertilization," *Fertility and Sterility* 38:673 (1982).

13. M. Wikland, L. Enk, L. Hamberger, "Transvesical and Transvaginal Approaches for the Aspiration of Follicles by Use of Ultrasound," *In Vitro Fertilization and Embryo Transfer*, ed. M. Seppala and R.G. Edwards. New York Academy of Sciences, vol. 442 (1985), 182.

14. H.W. Jones, A.A. Acosta, J. Garcia, "A Technique for the Aspiration of Oocytes from Human Ovarian Follicles," *Fertility and Sterility* 37:26 (1982).

15. M. Wikland, L. Nilsson, R. Hansson, L. Hamberger, P.O. Janson, "Collection of Human Oocytes by the Use of Sonography," *Fertility and Sterility* 39:603 (1983).

16. N.L. Freeman, A. Trounson, C. Kirby, "Cryopreservation of Human Embryos: Progress on the Clinical Use of the Technique in Human In Vitro Fertilization," *Journal of In Vitro Fertilization and Embryo Transfer* 3:53 (1986).

17. A. Trounson, "Preservation of Human Eggs and Embryos," *Fertility and Sterility* 46:1 (1986).

18. M. Seibel, "A New Era in Reproductive Technology: In Vitro Fertilization, Gamete Intrafallopian Transfer, and Donated Gametes and Embryos," *New England Journal of Medicine* 318:828 (1987).

19. The Ethics Committee of the American Fertility Society, "Ethical Considerations of the New Reproductive Technologies," *Fertility and Sterility* 46:Supplement 1 (September 1986).

JOHANNES HUBER, D.D.R.

Possible Modifications of Artificial Fertilization Techniques: Biological Considerations Which May Influence Theological Considerations

I shall attempt here to accomplish three goals concerning discussion of the in vitro fertilization process and other reproductive technologies. First, I shall investigate the possibility of modifying the methods of artificial fertilization used by the gynecologist so as to make them compatible with the directions in *Donum Vitae*. Second, I shall analyze, from the point of view of scientific evidence, the theological objections against artificial fertilization. Third, I shall describe some new methodologies in connection with in vitro fertilization. In addition, since the Vatican Instruction also discussed techniques of insemination, some ideas concerning this subject are presented from the biological and theological perspectives.

Insemination is defined as the insertion of sperm directly into the uterus of the wife by normal marital intercourse or by an assisted technique of catheterization of the cervix with insertion of the sperm previously collected by various techniques. Insemination may also be defined as the application of sperm from the husband directly onto the eggs harvested from the wife by surgical techniques and collected in a petri dish before these eggs are inserted back into the uterus. If the sperm is provided by the husband, the insemination is called homologous.

There are many indications for this therapy. They are, among others, *impotentia coeundi*, malformation of the male genital tract, and secondary anatomical changes produced by inflammatory diseases of the *cervix uteri*. The main indication for this treatment, however, is the condition of oligospermia, which is a reduced number and diminished mobility of sperm. By shortening the distance for the sperm to travel within the female genital tract—which is accomplished by the application of sperm directly into the cavity of the uterus—the chance for successful natural fertilization of eggs arises.

The Vatican Instruction strictly forbids this simple method of assisting fertilization even when the sperm is produced from the husband. There are two objections. First, it is pointed out that masturbation, even serving for diagnosis and therapy, is reprehensible and evil (IIB5). Second, an argument which has been brought forward again and again leading to the rejection of this method says that the generative and unitive aspects of the sexual act must be in one inseparable physical action (IIB5).

I am going to discuss below, from a scientific standpoint, these theological objections. I think, however, that the gynecologist should try his best, on the one hand, to search for modifications of present techniques to make assisted reproductive methods conform with the instructions contained in *Donum Vitae*, and on the other hand, to do this without making changes in the clinical effectiveness of these techniques. Therefore, some considerations are in order on ways to modify the technique of in vitro fertilization, the GIFT (Gamete Intrafallopian Transfer) procedure and other insemination techniques so that they are brought into conformity with the instructions in *Donum Vitae*. This is very important since the document does allow supportive medical techniques as long as they are performed in a manner which permits preservation of normal marital intercourse.

Some difficulties, indeed, may be found in the case of homologous insemination. We can try to obtain sperm which are produced during marital intercourse without resorting to masturbation by the husband. Thus, the possibility of a natural fertilization would not be excluded if after intercourse the physician obtains a sample of sperm from the vagina and then prepares it for insemination directly into the body of the uterus by catheter technique. This method is also very attractive from a medical point of view, as the quality (number and motility) of sperm obtained after intercourse is much better when analyzed than the quality of sperm obtained after masturbation. The use of a fenestrated condom has been employed previously. By this method, sperm could be collected from the pool in the condom and yet natural fertilization could never be excluded because in this procedure some sperm certainly could get into the genital tract of the wife and bring about fertilization in a natural way. Although this method has been accepted by the Roman moral theologians, it remains to be seen whether this type of assistance will be tolerated by the Roman authorities. This modified procedure is theologically problematic because conception can only be assumed after insemination; it cannot be assumed only after intercourse. A second objection to the above modification is a medical one. Since natural and normal physical intercourse is required, patients with *impotentia coeundi* cannot use this method.

In the case of the GIFT procedure, it is easier to modify the technique and to make it compatible with the instructions of *Donum Vitae*. Because this technique usually employs eggs obtained surgically and sperm produced without a marital sexual act, it is prohibited according to a strict interpretation of the document. But, the GIFT procedure can be modified—again by the fenestrated condom—so that marital intercourse does not have to be excluded and yet a supply of sperm can be obtained to mix with the eggs in the catheter. The mixture can be inserted back into the fallopian tube to allow insemination to take place naturally within the wife's body.

Human sperm survive in the female genital tract for forty-eight to fifty-six hours. This survival preserves their capacity for fertilization for at least twenty-four hours. The GIFT procedure could be modified in such a way that one day before the oocyte collection a normal marital intercourse is performed. The inseminated sperm ascends into the female genital tract and remains in the cervical crypts as well as in the oviducts. Sperm is still, twenty-four hours later, capable of fertilizing an oocyte. Within twenty-four hours after this intercourse, oocytes may be collected at a time determined by the endocrinologic and sonographic parameters. These can then be immediately transferred by surgical technique into the oviducts. Since sperm are already in this area, fertilization can take place. The usual indication for GIFT, namely, the idiopathic sterility from a disturbed vacuum mechanism of the fimbriae of the oviduct, may thus be overcome. It must be emphasized that in employing the above technique, the timing of intercourse and the timing of possible fertilization do not coincide. But during normal in vivo biological fertilization occurring after marital intercourse this is also true. The timing of marital intercourse and the timing of natural fertilization do not coincide. This will be discussed later.

Some difficulties in this technique do arise for the gynecologist when the oviducts are obstructed and marital coitus is regarded as a necessary condition for any treatment. In this case two possibilities, more hypothetical than real, come to mind. According to some reports, pregnancies have been achieved by transferring the oocyte into the proximal part of the fallopian tube by hysteroscopy immediately after collecting the eggs using the techniques of sonography or laparoscopy. A marital intercourse must also have been performed within the previous twenty-four hours. The critics of this method point out that during hysteroscopical intervention the endometrium is always damaged. Since many patients have no oviducts, the oocytes harvested can therefore only be deposited on an endometrium which is probably not sufficiently developed to sustain implantation.

For these reasons cryopreservation of oocytes would be helpful. Oocytes can be removed at one cycle, cryoconservated and transferred in the following cycle immediately after marital intercourse. The technique of cryopreservation of oocytes presents great difficulties. The question whether the spindle apparatus is destroyed by the freezing process is still a subject of controversy. On the other hand, there are several reports of successful pregnancies following cryoconservation of oocytes fertilized in the above fashion. The objection of the Sacred Congregation for the Doctrine of the Faith to the freezing of sperm was based on the fact that masturbation was required for the collection of sperm. This is not so in the case of oocyte collection. It remains debatable, however, whether the Congregation would have ethical questions about this medical intervention and manipulation.

The basic objection of the Congregation for the Doctrine of the Faith to artificial fertilization is that the coincidence of marital intercourse and the possibility of conception—that is, of "becoming a human being"—is interrupted. These doubts were well articulated at the 1976 Cracow Symposium, when the then Cardinal Wojtyla, now His Holiness, Pope John Paul II, invited several Polish scientists to discuss contraception and abortion.[1] At that time the arguments given constantly emphasized that fertilization must always be connected with the physical marital sexual act, viz., that the generative aspects and the unitive aspects of marital intercourse must always exist in a single act of physical marital sexual intercourse. This argument, given in a discussion about contraception, is now being applied to reproductive medicine where both the theological and biological complexities of animation are many and demand consideration.

God creates the soul but he only will do so, it was postulated at the Cracow Symposium, when couples carry out the physical progenitive act. This is the reason why the connection of "becoming a human being," on the one hand, and marital intercourse, on the other hand, is very rigidly sustained. But can this argument be maintained in the face of scientific evidence?

The method of in vitro fertilization has made it possible for the first time ever to study stages of fertilization in the human being. These studies confirm that fertilization is not an instantaneously chronological outcome connected with marital intercourse; it is also not connected to the actual migration and penetration of the spermatocyte into the oocyte. Fertilization can take place not only several days after sperm have been deposited in the female genital tract by marital intercourse, but also many hours after the penetration of the individual sperm into the oocyte. This has been pointed out many times. Fertilization within the egg itself is not an instantaneous process but requires at least twenty-four hours after the penetration of a single sperm into the oocyte. The two pronuclei, one from the sperm and one from the egg, do form reasonably quickly after penetration has taken place. These two pronuclei contain, respectively, the genetic information from the father and from the mother. The genetic composition of the new individual is constituted only after the fusion of these two pronuclei. But these paternal and maternal pronuclei containing the chromosomal material stay apart (and at some distance in the oocyte) for about twenty-four hours before they fuse. It is only after this time period has lapsed that the chromosomal material fuses. This process is called syngamy.

The arguments of the Cracow group ten years ago are based on—and this is documented in writing—the above scientifically described processes of fertilization, viz. that fertilization is not an instantaneous process but rather, a more continual one. Thus, the arguments are false on biological and theological grounds when they seek to support the often repeated dictum that the unitive and genitive aspects of marital intercourse must be connected directly in the one physical act. Even the reasons for objection to masturbation are difficult to sustain. The initial formulation which interpreted sperm as living beings (especially after the first microscopical investigation of sperm) is totally indefensible. These are not "homunculi" but at most only half-human cells containing only one-half of the normal number of human chromosomes. Also indefensible is the idea that masturbation carried out for reproduction only represents an egoistic action of the mind. The intention of an action does influence the morality of that action.

Note

1. Cardinal Karol Wojtyla, "Die personalistiche Konzeption des Menschen," in *Elternschaft und Menschenwürde Zur Problemmatic der Empfangnesregelung*, ed. E. Wenisch, G. Kaldenbach, and W.B. Skrzydlewski, O.P. (Vallendar-Schönstalt: Patris Verlag, 1984), 409.

III

MORAL-THEOLOGICAL FOUNDATIONS

JOHN P. LANGAN, S.J.

Moral Theology and Moral Teaching

The Catholic church in its moral teaching continually looks in two different directions. The first is the look within: to the community of the Catholic faithful who turn to church leadership for moral guidance in a changing world. In addressing this community, the church relies on Scripture and tradition. The second is the look outside: to the larger civil community that sets the legal and cultural context for ethical decisions and that is, at least intermittently, interested in moral issues. In carrying on dialogue and debate with this wider community, the church is under the necessity of articulating its position in rational terms or, at least, in terms that are common to itself and its dialogue partners.

The two pastoral letters of the U.S. Catholic bishops are examples of how the church in its social teaching wants to address a double audience—one Catholic, the other civic. In aiming at this double audience, the U.S. bishops are following the example of John XXIII, Paul VI, and John Paul II, who have addressed major encyclicals to "men and women of good will," as well as the precedent set by Vatican Council II in its great Constitution on the Church in the Modern World, *Gaudium et Spes*. In doing this, the church is not restricted to speaking on the classic social questions of economic justice and international peace. For many of the issues treated in the present Instruction and in other presentations of the church's teaching on biomedical ethics have public policy implications and raise questions that have to be answered in the form of public debate. At a more fundamental level there is a strong, inherent tendency in Catholic moral teaching to rely on reasoned argument in clarifying the demands of natural law and of the divine Creator of nature with respect to new situations. For in the words of St. Thomas Aquinas, "natural law is nothing other than the sharing in the Eternal Law by intelligent creatures."[1]

Both of the papers in this section, on the fundamental issues of moral theology in the Instruction, are concerned with the double direction in which Catholic moral teaching looks, even though they offer contrasting assessments of the Instruction itself. Professor Bruno Schüller, S.J., who teaches in the Catholic theological faculty of the University of Münster, treats the Instruction as largely paraenetic in character, that is, as an exhortation to those already convinced of the truth of the position being urged, rather than as an analysis and argument intended to be convincing to those who are skeptical.[2] John Haas, who holds a Ph.D. in moral theology from the Catholic University of America, and teaches at the Pontifical College Josephinum in Worthington, Ohio, sees the Instruction as offering "a reasoned exposition of basic human goods and values to be safeguarded and promoted." Whereas Schüller finds many of the arguments advanced in the Instruction to be question-begging or based on persuasive definitions,[3] Haas stresses primarily the contribution that the Instruction makes to the defense of two key values: the dignity of the human person and the dignity of procreation. Both Haas and Schüller are seriously concerned about the soundness of the arguments used in this area of moral theology. Both have been influenced by the analytic school of moral philosophy, and both reject naturalism in ethics, a metaethical view which argues from certain facts in nature to ethical conclusions and which has played a significant part in many traditional presentations of Catholic moral theology.[4]

Schüller and Haas, however, differ significantly in their assessments of technological intervention in the reproductive process. Schüller asks us to consider the possibility that medical interventions may have the characteristics of love and giving which the Instruction requires in actions that are to be the source of a new life. Haas does not dismiss artificial interventions as immoral simply on the ground of their artificiality, since that would be a form of ethical naturalism. But he is profoundly distrustful of the technological transformation or replacement of coitus. The Instruction itself insists repeatedly on the need for keeping technological interventions within moral limits. Haas makes it clear that in his view Catholic theology exalts the physicality of the human body and its sexual acts. But Schüller replies that the point of a couple's turning to technological intervention and specifically to homologous artificial insemination is not to replace or degrade sexual activity, but to remedy a defect in their own conjugal act, a defect which produces a de facto separation of intercourse and procreation.

This is the stage in the debate where we see most clearly the influence of earlier debates on moral norms and exceptions that have raged in both Protestant and Catholic theology over the last thirty years. For the justification of in vitro fertilization, if it is justifiable, is the justification of an action that is resorted to in order to remedy an otherwise irremediable situation. This exceptional character holds for reasons of cost, risk, and complexity even before one begins to consider moral objections to the procedure. The debate between those who would justify exceptions to concrete moral norms for proportionate reasons and those who hold that at least some norms must be acknowledged to be exceptionless is an ongoing battle among moral theologians and philosophers. Schüller himself is renowned as a particularly acute defender of the proportionalist position. Those who shaped and defend the Instruction hold the contrary view.

But it is worth observing that the Instruction itself increases the difficulty of the task for the absolutists or antiproportionalists. For the Instruction puts before its readers an attractive and persuasive model of the connections that should exist among marriage, sexual activity, procreation, and parenthood. For instance, it says:

The child has the right to be conceived, carried in the womb, brought into the world and brought up within marriage. It is through the secure and recognized relationship to his own parents that the child discovers his own identity and achieves his own proper human development.

The parents find in their child a confirmation of their reciprocal self-giving: the child is the living image of their love, the permanent sign of their conjugal union, the living and indissoluble concrete expression of their paternity and maternity.

By reason of the vocation and social responsibilities of the person, the good of the children and of the parents contributes to the good of civil society; the vitality and stability of society require that children come into the world within a family and that the family be firmly based on marriage.

This is a position that very few would want to challenge, and it offers a positive understanding of marriage and family that goes well beyond restrictive legalism. But the problem is that as the church offers a richer, more attractive model of marriage and family life, the difficulty of instantiating this model in practice increases. It is true that the model offers powerful motivating considerations that well may be helpful to families that are in difficulty. But fewer families, fewer marriages are likely to realize the model. The problem is both logical and sociological. On the logical side, the more positive elements one puts into the model, the more opportunities there are bound to be for falling short. On the sociological side, both in secularized, advanced, industrial societies and in the fragile economies and polities of the Third World, there are increasingly powerful pressures at work making it harder for larger and larger numbers of people to fit the model. The number of exceptions, the number of persons who cannot fit the model for many different reasons, is bound to increase. This presents the church with great pastoral problems, and it presents society with increasing numbers of people needing assistance in various ways. But it also challenges the church to assess the right and the wrong ways of coping with exceptional situations. This debate among moral theologians may help us to do this in a way that is both faithful and charitable.

Notes

1. St. Thomas Aquinas, *Summa Theologiae*, I-II, 91, 2c, tr. Thomas Gilby, O.P. (London: Blackfriars, 1966), 23.

2. On paraenesis, see the brief article by J.L. Houlden in *The Westminster Dictionary of Christian Ethics*, ed. James Childress and John Macquarrie (Philadelphia: Westminster Press, 1986), 448.

3. The classic discussion of persuasive definitions is in Charles L. Stevenson, *Ethics and Language*, (New Haven, Conn.: Yale University Press, 1944), 206-26.

4. A clear and judicious explanation of this term and its significance for moral epistemology, which is quite different from its meaning in metaphysics and theology, can be found in William Frankena, *Ethics*, 2d ed. (Englewood Cliffs, N.J.: Prentice-Hall, 1973), 97-102.

BRUNO SCHÜLLER, S.J.

Paraenesis and Moral Argument
in Donum Vitae

Before beginning, I will introduce myself by way of two preliminary remarks which may preclude certain misunderstandings. First, with regard to the fragmentary kind of commentary that I will make on the Instruction at issue, I am far from claiming that it—my commentary—is particularly important or even crucial. It will only show you how I, for one, am used to reading and analyzing any text on moral matters, irrespective of its author. Some might find my line of reading and analysis rather or even extremely pedantic. To them I can only reply: I am sorry, I can't help it; it's an incurable disease. Second, in the course of the last ten years I have come to realize more and more that I personally would not be able to survive either as a philosopher or as a theologian without the aid of both irony and a sense of humor. I am happy that about two years ago I happened to come across an ally, Krister Stendahl, formerly professor of New Testament at Harvard, now Lutheran Bishop of Stockholm, Sweden. In the preface to his book *Paul among Jews and Gentiles*, he writes: "It is my conviction that theology is too serious to allow humans to think theologically without playfulness and irony... There is a theological necessity of irony—and its nobler cousin humor—as a safeguard against idolatry."[1] *Mutatis mutandis*, I must own that as a moral theologian I have a regrettably diminished sense of responsibility. That is, I feel responsible for clear thinking and impeccable reasoning in moral matters, even though I am fully alive to the truth that *Non in dialectica complacuit Deo salvum facere populum suum.*

Last year, in the week of Corpus Christi, I attended in Barcelona a closed conference of mostly continental medical experts and moral theologians. One question we had to grapple with, in a way suggested by Cardinal Martini, concerned the teaching of what is usually called the authentic magisterium of the church in moral matters: to what extent does this teaching have the character of paraenesis, that is, of moral exhortation and *not* of normative ethics in the technical sense of this term? The question, while admittedly of great consequence, appears to be almost impossible to answer, when asked in this general form. The pronouncements of Pope Pius XII as *magister authenticus*, collected in a German edition, amount to three sturdy volumes. Who can claim to have read them all so carefully that he is in a position to assess their *genus litterarium*? And even these volumes contain only the most important part of the pronouncements of the *magisterium authenticum* as discharged between 1939 and 1958. What are nineteen years in the history of the magisterium?

There is, however, an easy remedy for this problem. We have only to make up our minds to be modest and to confine ourselves to some specific pronouncement of the magisterium, for instance to *Humanae Vitae*. To what extent is this encyclical moral exhortation rather than normative ethics? Fortunately, I find myself able to quote an answer to this question, which is given by someone who wholeheartedly agrees with the encyclical. A Swiss priest and philosopher, Martin Rhonheimer, published a voluminous dissertation in which he takes to task almost the whole community of contemporary German-speaking moral theologians. Although there is hardly anyone who finds favor in his eyes, he is in agreement with Germain Grisez and John Finnis. In his argument, he quotes the crucial thesis of *Humanae Vitae*, that there is an "inseparable connection willed by God and incapable of being broken by man on his own initiative, between the two meanings of the conjugal act, the unitive meaning and the procreative meaning."[2] In a footnote to this quotation, Rhonheimer observes: "To be sure, that this connection of the two meanings corresponds to the will of God must be justified by way of an anthropological and ethical analysis. Such an analysis is not to be found in *Humanae Vitae*; for *Humanae Vitae* is an encyclical and not a treatise of moral theology."[3] If Rhonheimer is right, then *Humanae Vitae* simply asserts the moral wrongness of artificial contraception and does not justify the assertion by giving and explaining the reason or reasons for this moral verdict. I am of the opinion that Rhonheimer is right; indeed, this is one of the extremely few points on which I agree with him. If it is the case that the encyclical offers no reasoning for its moral judgment, how are we to account for the fact that it is a rather lengthy document? The encyclical makes abundant use of a stylistic device, often characteristic of liturgical and paraenetic discourse: linguistic variation and amplification. An example of this linguistic device at its very best can be found in Thomas à Kempis' *Imitation of Christ*, book 3, chapter 54: "Of the Different Motions of Nature and Grace."

"Nature is unwilling," Thomas says, "to be mortified, bridled or overcome, to be under subjection or to accept obedience... But grace studieth self-mortification, withstands sensuality, seeketh to be in subjection... Nature laboureth for her own advantage, and always considereth what gain she may reap at the expense of another, but grace considereth not what is profitable and advantageous unto herself, but rather may be for the good of the many." Is there anyone who can deny or doubt the truth of these propositions? No one can, provided he is in command of the moral vocabulary employed by Thomas. The word-pair 'nature and grace,' as used by Thomas, is equivalent to the Pauline word-pair 'flesh and spirit,' *sarx kai pneuma*. Recall that in Galatians, chapter 5, a catalogue of vices is introduced by the phrase: the works of flesh; a catalogue of virtues is introduced by the expression: the fruit of the spirit. If you keep this in mind, you will not fail to notice that in the following passage from the above-mentioned chapter Thomas explains the motions of nature by describing various vices and the motions of grace by expounding various virtues.

Let us now return to *Humanae Vitae*. In 1969 and 1970, I studied and analyzed this encyclical with painstaking care and noted that the encyclical *Humanae Vitae* seems at first glance to contain, under the numerals 11-13, an argumentative part (= normative ethics). But a thorough examination and analysis of the text discloses that appearances are deceptive. The text does nothing but, in the manner of paraenesis, again and again vary the one sentence: the use of artificial contraceptives is illicit. In *Humanae Vitae* this sentence is, by and large, put in the positive form: The conjugal act must always combine the *significatio unitatis* and the *significatio procreationis*. The term *significatio procreationis* is implicitly defined in a way that only artificial contraception, not the so-called "rhythm method," is excluded. In this positive formulation, the encyclical varies the expressions *significatio unitatis*, *significatio procreationis* and the *modale copula* 'must be' or 'ought to be'. This is not difficult to verify. One has only to draw up lists of synonyms or quasi-synonyms, according to the rubrics: (1) equivalents of *significatio unitatis*; (2) equivalents of *significatio procreationis*; (3) equivalents of 'ought to be' in the moral sense. With regard to the last rubric, one has to call to mind how rich our moral vocabulary is in quasi-synonyms of the expressions 'morally right' and 'wrong'. If one chooses from every list one single term and puts it into the sentences of the encyclical, thus avoiding all synonymous expressions, the fact simply cannot be overlooked: what takes place is solely the variation and modification of a single sentence. This observation is not intended as criticism of the encyclical, but rather, serves to identify the text contained under numerals 11-13 as paraenesis.

In bringing these observations to bear on the Instruction on Respect for Human Life in Its Origin and on the Dignity of Procreation, we must ask, to what extent has the Instruction the character of moral exhortation? In the document's conclusion, all those who can exercise a positive influence are invited "to ensure that, in the family and in society, due respect is accorded to life and love." Is anyone willing to deny that due respect must be accorded to life and love? The church, it is said, "hopes that all will understand the incompatibility between recognition of the dignity of the human person and contempt for life and love, between faith in the living God and the claim to decide arbitrarily the origin and fate of a human being." I cannot quite see why it is said of the church that she *hopes* for such an understanding. Can the church not be reassured? Nobody in command of the language of morals can fail to understand the asserted incompatibility, for it is analytically evident. Incidentally, to decide *arbitrarily* the fate of a human being seems to be not only incompatible with faith in the living God, but also with the moral point of view. Possibly, in the vocabulary of the Instruction, the expressions 'faith in the living God' and 'moral point of view' are semantically interchangeable as in religious language the terms 'moral demand' and 'will of God'. Exhortatory utterances, if they are, against their own intention, read as informative utterances, usually prove to be analytically evident. A paradigm case can be found in the fifth commandment of the Decalogue: Thou shalt do no murder.

Obviously, the Instruction is not only moral exhortation. It gives answers to some serious moral questions: What respect is due to the human embryo? Is artificial fertilization morally right or wrong? The answers of the Instruction are unambiguous. It is trivially true that anyone who regards the answer to a question as correct, implicitly asks for universal assent. Could it be the case that the Instruction has this assent in mind, when hoping that "all will understand the incompatibility between recognition of the dignity of the human person and contempt for life and love"? Suppose somebody considers homologous artificial insemination as morally right. Does he, by thinking so, disclose his contempt for love? Among moral theologians two varieties of a *reductio ad absurdum* are very popular, the *reductio ad improbitatem* and the *reductio ad impietatem*. Could it possibly be the case that *loco citato* the Instruction also makes use of these devices of refutation?

Once again, the answers of the Instruction are unambiguous. But are they presented as the result of rigorous moral reasoning? Let us have a closer look. In the fourth part of the introduction, the Instruction reminds us of two "fundamental criteria for the moral judgment" on the questions at issue. First, "the inviolability of the innocent human being's right to life from the moment of conception until death." Second, that "the transmission of human life is entrusted by nature to a personal and conscious act and as such is subject to the all-holy laws of God: immutable and inviolable laws which must be recognized and observed." Are these two criteria something like moral principles that enable us to pass the correct judgment on the questions at issue? I doubt it. They are already the answers to the questions at issue. Suppose I am right in that. What have we to expect from the rest of the Instruction? A justification of these criteria? Or rather an analytically evident explanation and elaboration of the two criteria laid down in the preface? Incidentally, the linguistically redundant formulation of the second criterion is striking: "The transmission of human life...is subject to the all-holy laws of God; immutable and inviolable laws which must be recognized and observed." That God's inviolable laws must be observed and not violated, seems to be true by definition. Some lines later the Instruction states that "what is technically possible is not for that very reason morally admissible." When I first read this sentence, I could not help smiling. I do not know how often I have come across this maxim with German moral theologians. All of them accept it unhesitatingly. Small wonder! Its rejection is equivalent to a rejection of the moral point of view. All the same, I admit, all of us are in need of being reminded of this truism, since all of us are constantly in need of moral exhortation.

The main part of the Instruction strikes me as somehow odd in its structure. Take the paragraphs on heterologous artificial fertilization. The headline of the first paragraph consists in the question: "Why must human procreation take place in marriage?" (IIA1). The answer is given about thirty-five lines down. The second paragraph follows with the headline: "Does heterologous artificial fertilization conform to the dignity of the couple and to the truth of marriage?" What could be the point of this second question? Is it not simply redundant? If only in marriage is procreation morally right, then heterologous artificial insemination of necessity must be morally wrong, that is, incompatible with the dignity of the couple and the truth of marriage. Incidentally, are the terms 'the dignity of the couple' and 'the truth of marriage' not semantically interchangeable? At any rate, the Instruction uses about fifteen lines to answer the second question: Heterologous artificial fertilization is contrary to the dignity of the spouses, contrary to the unity of marriage, and so on. The whole passage ends in this way: "These reasons *lead* [!] to a negative moral judgment concerning heterologous artificial fertilization: It is morally illicit (IIA2). A very odd phrase, indeed. The incompatibility of a certain course of action with the dignity of the agent is a reason that leads to a negative moral judgment on this course of action. The paragraphs on homologous artificial fertilization have exactly the same structure. The outcome of the first paragraph is that "the procreation of a person must be the fruit and result of married love" (IIB4b). If this is settled, then it is hardly necessary to explain in two more paragraphs that in vitro fertilization and artificial insemination are morally wrong. If it is made clear that we must speak the truth, is it then still meaningful to enlarge on the moral wrongness of telling lies? It may be meaningful, provided that the purpose pursued is moral exhortation.

Let us now turn to the part of the Instruction that treats homologous artificial insemination. I shall begin with the first line and go on for a while, sentence by sentence, in the way of a *lectio currens*. In the first question: "What connection is required from the moral point of view between procreation and the conjugal act?," we are reminded of the church's teaching (*Humanae Vitae*). This teaching affirms again "the inseparable connection willed by God." The second sentence repeats the first in different words: "Indeed, by its intimate structure, the conjugal act, while most closely uniting husband and wife, capacitates them for the generation of new lives, according to laws inscribed in the very being of man and woman." I skip the third sentence as irrelevant for our purpose. The fourth sentence: "By safeguarding both these essential aspects, the unitive and the procreative, the conjugal act preserves in its fullness the sense of true mutual love and its ordination toward man's exalted vocation to parenthood." is again a purely linguistic variation of the first sentence.

In the next three passages the same is said per *modum negationis*: Artificial contraception and artificial fertilization dissociate the inseparable meaning of the conjugal act; hence they are morally illicit. Up to this point, we are given an assertion, but no intrinsic reason why this assertion is true. So what is exactly the reason for the inseparable meanings of the conjugal act? Although the following passages also fail to provide this reason, there is, however, a very revelatory inference. The document states that "the origin of a human person is the result of an act of giving. The one conceived must be the fruit of his parents' love. He cannot be desired or conceived as the product of an intervention of medical or biological techniques; that would be equivalent to reducing him to an object of scientific technology" (IIB4c).

I will admit that the origin of a human person has to be the result of an act of giving, but is there no other act of giving beyond the conjugal act? What disqualifies the intervention of medical techniques as having the character of an act of giving? I agree that the one conceived must be the fruit of his parents' love, but again, is the parents' love simply identical with the conjugal act? Whatever they do disinterestedly for the benefit of a potential child, they do out of love. And the benefit is the fruit of love. There is in the Instruction a somewhat contestable sequence of designations of the conjugal act. First, the conjugal act is an act by which the couple mutually *express* their self-gift; in this sense it is a kind of speech-act, the meaning of which is love. Second, the conjugal act is called an act of love. Third, the conjugal act is simply designated as love. Obviously, it is not possible to say that what is not the fruit of the conjugal act (as a specific speech-act of love) is for this reason not the fruit of an act of love (and consequently not the fruit of love). But to all appearances, the Instruction makes this inference. To the Instruction, the dignity of procreation, that is, the exclusion of homologous artificial fertilization, seems to be equivalent to the "due respect accorded to love."

There is a further difficulty with the manner in which the Instruction speaks of the conjugal act as an act of mutual love. Even spouses as spouses can be sinners, can act out of pure self-love or selfishness. Therefore, it is possible that in their conjugal intercourse they use each other as a means for their own self-interest. What have we to call a child procreated by an act of this description? Is it the fruit of two egoisms united? It can perhaps be insisted that even in a case like this, the marital act, its objective structure, remains the speech-act whose meaning is genuine love. But I doubt that we are much better off if we make this assumption. For in this case, we would have to call the child the fruit of a conjugal lie.

Presumably, difficulties of this kind arise because the Instruction characterizes the marital act not solely as morally right, but also as morally good when, without qualification, it refers to it as an act of mutual love and self-giving. This procedure has still another consequence. We have to distinguish artificial insemination from procreation through the marital act. What alone can be the *principium divisionis*, if from the start the conjugal act is introduced as an act of mutual love? Only this mutual love, its presence or absence. Thus, absence of love must be the *differentia specifica* of artificial insemination. By a logical division of this sort, artificial insemination shows up as morally doomed from the start.

Hence the question: how must we characterize the marital act, if referring exclusively to its moral rightness? There was a time when our own tradition used for this purpose the term '*debitum conjugale*' or 'marriage debt'. If we pick up this term, we can reword the claim of the Instruction as follows: "The one conceived must be the fruit of the act that constitutes his or her parents' 'marriage debt'." The claim, if worded like that, sounds considerably less impressive. As an alternative, perhaps we could resort to the distinction between love as benevolence and love as beneficence. Feeding the hungry is an act of beneficence, even though my reason for doing so might be morally highly objectionable, viz., because it has nothing at all to do with benevolence, the attitude of disinterested love. Accordingly, referring to the conjugal act solely insofar as it is morally right, we could call it an act of mutual beneficence. The claim of the Instruction, correspondingly reformulated, runs as follows: The one conceived must be the fruit of the conjugal act, as an act of mutual beneficence. A sentence that is not particularly impressive.

What is conjugal love? Allow me to quote a short passage from C.S. Lewis in response to this question. "Most of our ancestors were married off in early youth to partners chosen by their parents on grounds that had nothing to do with Eros. They went to the act with no other 'fuel,' so to speak, than plain animal desire. And they did right; honest Christian husbands and wives, obeying their fathers and mothers, discharging to one another their 'marriage debt,' and bringing up families in the fear of the Lord."[4] Were the couples to whom Lewis refers, *ex supposito* not really motivated by agape in the Christian sense? But what will be the exact meaning of the Instruction's rich love vocabulary, when applied to such couples?

According to the Instruction, we remember, homologous artificial fertilization would be equivalent to "reducing the child to an object of scientific technology." This way of expressing moral disapproval seems to be based on a linguistic variation of Kant's second formula of the Categorical Imperative: "Act in such a way that you always treat humanity, whether in your own person or in the person of any other, never simply as a means, but always at the same time as an end." As is well known, for Kant, using someone as a mere means is the same as using someone as a mere thing, as an object, as a *Sache*. Now, I would like to learn what it is that disqualifies the agents of medical techniques of artificial fertilization from being seen as treating the humanity in the person of the child as an end in itself. Incidentally, when I read the oppositions: the child, "the fruit of love," not "the product of an intervention of medical technique," I cannot help being reminded of the use of so-called persuasive definition, or of question-begging nouns.

With regard to the second formula of the Categorical Imperative, Sir David Ross observes: "It has in fact great homiletic value; it is a means of edification rather than of enlightenment."[5] Possibly this homiletic value makes it understandable why many moralists, philosophers as well as theologians, so often (if I am permitted to judge from my own experience) improperly appeal to this formula. Kant himself used it in order to prove that the death penalty is an absolute moral demand. Concerning the Catholic doctrine of the indissolubility of marriage as a sacrament, R. Fletcher writes: This is "clearly to treat human individuals not as ends in themselves but as means only—in this case as means to correct observance of religious law, or even divine law. But if God exists, and is a moral being, he could not possibly want it so."[6]

It may be useful at this point to engage in some historical reminiscences. In 1939 and again in 1946, Fr. G. Kelly wrote articles on (homologous) artificial insemination. Both times his conclusion was the solidly probable licitness of this procedure. He mentions that moral theologians like Génicot-Salsmans, Iorio, Noldin-Schmitt, Payen and Vermeersch advocate the same view. But in 1946, F. Hürth, the very influential advisor of Pope Pius XII, published in the *Nouvelle Revue Théologique* his article "La Fécondation Artificielle,"[7] strongly rejecting this method. He seems to have made a considerable impression on many of his fellow moral theologians. At any rate, in 1949, in *Theological Studies*, Kelly reviewed four recently published papers, all of them disapproving of artificial insemination. Kelly concluded his review with the following remark: "On two previous occasions I have defended the probable licitness of such insemination. I should be blind not to see the growing trend against this opinion, and unreasonable not to respect it. Though not convinced by the arguments, I am certainly impressed by them. Since nothing would be gained by continuing this debate, I am retiring into a more peaceful (and perhaps more secure) atmosphere."[8] On September 29 of the same year, Pius XII, as *magister authenticus*, pronounced artificial insemination to be morally wrong, and explained: "Qu'on ne l'oublie pas: seule la procréation d'une nouvelle vie selon la volonté et le plan du Créateur porte avec elle, à un degré étonnant de perfection, la réalisation des buts poursuivis. Elle est, à la fois, conformé à la nature corporelle et spirituelle et à la dignité des époux, au développement normal et heureux de l'enfant."[9] F. Hürth published a commentary on the Pope's allocution in the *Periodica*, September 15th.[10] Was the commentary ready for print two weeks before the Pope delivered the allocution?[11]

The explanation given by the Pope is clearly reminiscent of the vocabulary employed by the present Instruction. To be sure, it does not amount to any justification of the moral verdict on artificial insemination. If only procreation through the marital act is right, then only this procreation can be "selon la volonté et le plan du Créateur" as well as "conformé à la nature...et dignité des epoux." But why is only this kind of procreation "selon la volonté du Créateur?" The reasoning on which this assertion is based can be studied in the above-mentioned article by Hürth on "artificial insemination." After enlarging on the physiology and psychology of the conjugal act, strongly emphasizing procreation as its end, Hürth concludes: "Our whole reasoning proves not merely that nature has shown how to serve the human species by procreating offspring, but also that nature admits of no other procedure." "Indeed," writes Hürth, "it would be absurd, if nature provided a means or a different one of their own invention. Nature does not tolerate withint itself contradictions of this kind." Hürth finds "la volonté de la nature inscrite dans les organs et leur fonction."[12] (Volonté de la nature = volonté du Créateur.)

Does the Instruction think so as well? Probably it does, even though it is more delicate in its formulations: (1) "The transmission of human life is entrusted by nature to a personal and conscious act" (Intro. 4). (2) "By its intimate structure, the conjugal act, while most closely uniting husband and wife, capacitates them for the generation of new lives, according to laws inscribed in the very being of man and woman" (IIB4a).

But why are husband and wife tempted to have recourse to artificial insemination? Is it not, above all, because the transmission of human life is *not* entrusted to their own conjugal act by nature, that their own conjugal act does *not* capacitate them for the generation of new lives, that the laws inscribed in their very being are ineffective or defective? Is it inconceivable that God has provided man with reason and understanding also so that he, by himself, may endeavor to find out how to succeed when natural measures prove a failure?

The way the Instruction describes or rather characterizes such human endeavors is worth noticing. "The generation of a child must...be the fruit of that mutual giving which is realized in the conjugal act wherein the spouses cooperate as servants and not as masters in the work of the Creator" (IIB6). It is plain that whoever has recourse to artificial insemination arrogates to himself the part of master, whereas a human being's part can only be that of the servant of God, his Creator. "Homologous IVF and ET is brought about outside the bodies of the couple through actions of third parties whose competence and technical activities determine the success of the procedure. Such fertilization entrusts the life and identity of the embryo into the power of doctors and biologists and establishes the domination over the origin and destiny of a human person" (IIB5). There can be no doubt what the meaning of these propositions is. I hope, however, you will forgive me that I cannot resist the temptation to rephrase this characterization. Artificial insemination appears to be required by the so-called *principium subsidiaritatis.* "Ought implies can." Only those can be morally obliged to help, who have the skill and competence necessary for help. It is true, in the case of artificial insemination, that the life and identity of the embryo is entrusted to the power of doctors and biologists. But his power determines exactly the measure of the moral responsibility of doctors and biologists. And from the moral point of view, the purpose of their domination over a human person can only be the well-being of this human person as an end it itself. *Servire regnare est.*

The Instruction speaks in rather derogatory terms of "biological techniques," "scientific technology" and "technical efficiency," insofar as they characterize artificial insemination. "Conception in vitro"—we are told—"is the result of the technical actions which presides over fertilization" (IIB5). There is no denying this fact. But is it not the case that nature too can entrust the transmission of life to husband and wife only by providing certain "techniques," if I am permitted this term. St. Thomas Aquinas, in *Summa Contra Gentiles*, III 126 states *"quod non omnis carnalis commixtio sit peccatum."* He expresses himself in the following way:

> Cum membra corporis sint quaedam animae instrumenta[!], cuisulibet membri finis est usus eius, sicut et cuiuslibet alterius instrumenti[!]. Quorundam autem membrorum corporis usus est carnalis commixtio. Carnalis igitur commixtio est finis quorundam membrorum corporis. Id autem quod est finis aliquarum naturalium rerum non potest esse secundum se malum, quia ea quae naturaliter sunt, ex divina providentia ordinantur ad finem.

Thomas characterized the sexul organs as instruments and the conjugal act as the proper use of these instruments, as the purpose these instruments are devised for, by Divine Providence, that is, by God the Creator. As such, God is sometimes called by early Greek theologians "technites," which Lampe renders as "architect of the universe and supreme artist," more specifically as "designer of the human body."[13] After these reminiscences I would like simply to ask the question: what is wrong with "biological techniques," "technical efficiency" and "technical action," when the transmission of human life is at stake? Indubitably, the techniques devised by human beings strike us as utterly crude, if compared with the conjugal act, devised by the supreme wisdom of Divine Providence. But what if the conjugal act fails to procreate new life?

The Instruction does not object to medical intervention, "when it seeks to assist the conjugal act either in order to facilitate its performance or in order to enable it to achieve its objective once it has been performed." An intervention like that "respects the dignity of persons" (IIB7). Therefore it is understandable that some moral theologians have tried to clarify the distinction between such an intervention and artificial insemination. I shall quote anonymously: (1) "Nec demonstratur agi certo de inseminatione artificiali, si incitur versus uterum sperma ex ipso acto conjugali re tenti in cochleari immisso vel in 'condom' perforato. Actus autem vere condomisticus (condom clausum) vix justificari videtur per subsequentem injectionem spermatis, quae ergo esset inseminatio artificialis." (2) "Opus naturae tunc solum interrumpitur si instrumentum cum spermate extrahitur e vagina ut iterum inducatur." When the conjugal act is performed under circumstances implicitly mentioned in these quotations, in what exact sense does it "preserve in its fullness the sense of true mutual love?" Would it not be more to the point to say that under such circumstances husband and wife discharge to one another their "marriage debt"? Besides, provided that the considerations of the cited moral theologians are to the point, it is sometimes very difficult to make out whether "the spouses cooperate as servants...in the work of the Creator" or rather "as masters."

I allow, my last observation is not quite fair. Expressions characteristic of and appropriate for religious moral exhortation cannot simply be transferred to the sphere of normative ethics which, above all as applied ethics, cannot avoid the prose of casuistry. Such a transference can only be correct if it is at the same time a translation. A task still to be performed, and one which certainly will take considerable time, is the translation of the present Instruction into the prose of normative ethics. One thing is beyond any doubt. As to length, the translated text will be only a fragment of the present text. The degree to which the Instruction excels in paraenetic wordiness is in fact quite extraordinary, though neither uncommon nor unequalled among modern theologians. From experience, I know that wordy theologians very often are not aware of their wordiness. Misled by the erroneous notion of *"unum nomen—unum nominatum,"* they do not ask themselves in their thinking and reading whether two words or phrases are only different ways of saying the same thing. For instance, there are exegetes who take it for granted that the

Golden Rule, as used in Matthew and Luke, and the commandment of love (Lv 19:18) are two different moral principles. And to all appearances there are theologians and philosophers who do not realize the above-mentioned richness of moral vocabulary in synonyms of the moral value-words 'good and bad', 'right and wrong'.

Permit me to quote just two pairs of sentences form the Instruction:

> (1) "if the technical means facilitates the conjugal act or helps it to reach its natural objectives, it can be morally acceptable" (IIB6).
> (2) "A medical intervention respects the dignity of persons when it seeks to assist the conjugal act..." (IIB7).

Are these two sentences equivalent? Or have we to read: this procedure is morally acceptable, *because* it respects the dignity of persons?

> (1) "If... the procedure were to replace the conjugal act, it is morally illicit" (IIB6).
> (2) "It sometimes happens that a medical procedure technologically replaces the conjugal act... In this case the medical act is not, as it should be, at the service of conjugal union but rather appropriates to itself the procreative function and thus contradicts the dignity and the inalienable rights of the spouses and of the child to be born" (IIB7).

Are the two sentences in the given context equivalent, different only in their explicitness? Or should we say that the reasons given in the second proposition justify the moral verdict of the first proposition? I could imagine that someone has the impression that raising questions like that amounts to pure hair-splitting. It is well known that the fallacy of begging the question occurs nowhere so often as in the area of ethics.

The question just raised must be answered in order to avoid this fallacy. The limits of space make it impossible for me to *lege artis* answer the question merely to ask it, and so I must confine myself to giving some hints. Kant's second formulation of the

Catergorical Imperative can be used as a definition of the moral point of view. As Kant puts it, a person has absolute value, insofar as that person is an end in itself. That constitutes the dignity of a person. Therefore, 'to act as one ought to act' means 'to treat persons as persons, to respect their dignity'. So it seems obvious, the expressions 'a morally right act' and 'an act respecting the dignity of persons' are interchangeable. We have to read the first pair of sentences: this procedure is morally acceptable, *in other words*, it respects the dignity of persons. The phrase 'dignity of the spouses' has be to be defined by the duties and rights of the spouses. It is the abstract noun corresponding to the vocational and entitling names 'spouses' or 'husband and wife'. Thus the expression 'this course of action contradicts the dignity and inalienable rights of the spouses' is simply equivalent to: 'this course of action treats spouses in a way they ought not to be treated'. It is only a different formulation and not a justification of the moral judgment that this course of action is morally illicit. These hints may suffice. The translation of the Instruction into the prose of normative ethics cannot be done without a list of all the synonyms of the Instruction's vocabulary, at least kept in mind. By the way, there is no reason to object to the use of synonyms. As Stephen Ullmann observes: "Aristotle's claim that 'synonyms are useful to the poet' was, if anything, an understatement...choice and variation, if discreetly handled, are not merely useful: they are indispensable to any style worthy of that name."[14]

I will conclude with a last crucial question: is an appeal to Divine Providence legitimate in the area of normative ethics? We are told in the fourth part of the Introduction to *Donum Vitae* that "the transmission of human life is entrusted by *nature* to a personal and conscious act." Who or what is nature that it would be able to entrust something to someone: It is the work of the Creator! So it is the Creator who entrusts something to someone. But how do we know that? I think it advisable to clarify the point of this question by using an amusing example from Psalm 104. The psalmist praises God the Creator who brings bread out of the earth and wine to gladden men's hearts. Islam too believes in Divine Providence. Would it for that reason agree with the psalmist? I doubt it. Perhaps Islam would insist that God brings out of the earth only grapes, *not* wine: that wine is a product of man, the result of a misuse of God's gift, of the innocent grapes. The specific way we attribute something to Divine Providence depends on the value judgment we pass on this something.

Let us return to the serious question at issue. No doubt, the conjugal act is a morally right act. Therefore, it is true that "the transmission of human life is entrusted by nature, i.e. by God" to this act. But under what condition are we entitled to qualify this assertion by saying: the transmission of human life is entrusted by nature, i.e. by God *exclusively* to the conjugal act? Under the condition that through a logically antecedent argument it is made sure that homologous artificial insemination is morally wrong. In other words, we are not doing normative ethics, but a specifically theological kind of metaethics, when appealing to Divine Providence or to God as Creator and Redeemer. Understandably enough, the Instruction takes such a kind of metaethics for granted and very frequently calls it to mind. One instance: "God, who is love and life, has inscribed in man and woman the vocation to share in a special way in his mystery of personal communion and in his work as Creator and Father" (Intro. 3). Is there any Christian who is willing to question or to deny that God is love and life? And who will make bold to assert that moral theologians like A. Vermeersch or G.Kelly did not grasp the bearing of their faith in God as love and life, when arguing for the moral licitness of homologous artificial insemination? In the assertion just cited, the Instruction takes the moral wrongness of this procedure for an issue already settled and only reminds us of the theological dimension of this moral verdict. The plausibility, however, of this theological dimension must not be regarded as something like a convincing argument for the truth of this moral judgment. A Christian who is sure that there is a very strong case for homologous artificial insemination has not the slightest difficulty in giving his moral appraisal an equally convincing theological dimension. In short, a translation of the Instruction into the prose of normative ethics will also have to discard all the metaethical explanations of more judgments which are more or less taken for granted.

Now, let us suppose counterfactually that we have the text translated into the prose of normative ethics before us, at least that part which deals with homologous artificial insemination and in vitro fertilization. What would the text be like? It is not unlikely that it would consist only in a single sentence: both procedures are morally unacceptable. As is well known, formerly it it was not uncommon for the Holy Office to answer questions in this highly concise way. Compare Dz. 3788: Decretum S. Officii, 21.2 1940. Question: "An licita sit directa sterilizatio sive perpetua sive temporanea, sive viri sive mulieris." Answer: "Negative, et quidem prohiberi lege naturae, eamque, quod sterilizationem eugenicam attinet, Decreto 21.3 1931 reprobatam iam esse." As a scholar, one will hardly be inclined now to appreciate answers given in this fashion. Hannah Arendt, however, observes: "Authority... is incompatible with persuasion which presupposes equality and works through a process of argumentation. Where arguments are used, authority is left in abeyance."[15] I share Hannah Arendt's view. Only I ask myself whether at least sometimes authority would not act wisely by leaving its authority in abeyance and by having recourse to a process of argumentation.

Notes

1. Krister Stendahl, *Paul among Jews and Gentiles* (Philadelphia: Fortress Press, 1983), 2.
2. M. Rhonheimer, *Natur als Grundlage der Moral* (Innsbruck: Tyrolia-Verlag, 1987), 291.
3. Ibid., 28n.
4. C.S. Lewis, *The Four Loves* (London: G. Bles, 1960), 132.
5. W.D. Ross, *Kant's Ethical Theory* (Oxford: Clarendon Press, 1969), 55.
6. R. Fletcher, *The Family and Marriage in Britain* (Harmondsworth: Pelican Books, 1973), 244.
7. F. Hürth, "La Fécondation Artificielle," *Nouvelle Revue Théologique* 68 (1946):402-26.
8. G. Kelly, "Current Theology: Notes on Moral Theology," *Theological Studies* 10 (1949):113-14.
9. Pius XII, "Medical Ethics" (29 September 1949), *The Catholic Mind* 48 (1950):251.
10. F. Hürth, "Commentary on Pius XII's allocution, 'Medical Ethics'," *Periodica* 38 (1949):279-95.
11. F. Hürth, "La Fécondation Artificielle," 415.
12. Ibid., 413.
13. G.W.H. Lampe, ed., *A Patristic Greek Lexicon* (Oxford: Clarendon Press, 1978), 1393.
14. Stephen Ullman, *Semantics* (Oxford: Oxford University Press, 1977), 155.
15. Hannah Arendt, *Between Past and Future* (Harmondsworth: Penguin Books, 1977), 93.

JOHN M. HAAS, Ph.D.

The Natural and the Human
in Procreation

The discusions we are undertaking take place in a specific context, namely, the faith community known as the Roman Catholic Church. All of us are Catholics attempting to address difficult moral issues as men and women of faith who have certain shared beliefs. One of those beliefs distinctive to us as Catholics is the conviction that faith and reason are not incompatible; grace builds upon nature, it does not destroy it; Catholic moral teaching can, perhaps with some difficulty, be understood and appreciated in the light of natural reason. This is important to keep in mind because otherwise another Catholic belief which bears mentioning might be construed as anti-intellectual.

We Catholics also believe that the church has a particular competence to teach in the area of morals as well as faith so that Christians can know not only what they ought to believe, but also how they ought to behave to be pleasing to God. Even short of the exercise of infallibility, the magisterium is a sure guide in the area of belief and conduct. One reads in the Dogmatic Constitution of the Church of the Second Vatican Council:[1]

> the faithful ... are obliged to submit to their bishops' decision, made in the name of Christ, in matters of faith and morals, and to adhere to it with a ready and respectful allegiance of mind. This loyal submission of the will and intellect must be given, in a special way, to the authentic teaching authority of the Roman Pontiff, even when he does not speak 'ex cathedra' in such wise, indeed, that his supreme teaching authority be acknowledged with respect ...

The magisterium, of course, does not claim to have all the answers to every question of morality which might arise. In fact, the Catholic for the most part makes moral decisions throughout his life without reference to magisterial teaching. Yet Christians do have the benefit of such teaching to assist them "on their journey towards eternal beatitude."[2] And when the magisterium goes out of its way to address a moral issue, the presumption of truth will rest with its teaching so that one can follow it and always have moral certitude that he will not act in a way displeasing to God.[3] However, it is still the Catholic's responsibility to be quite clear about what a given magisterial document actually says, what degree of assent ought to be given to various propositions contained in it, and what is open for further development.[4] This paper will prescind from any consideration of the degree of magisterial authority attached to the Instruction under consideration.

Even the most solemnly taught moral doctrine of the church is usually presented through some argumentation. There are different ways in which magisterial documents themselves have made their own cases, some effectively and others less so. This became very apparent to me as I grappled personally with the magisterial teaching on the immorality of contraception. I had been raised a Protestant and had considered contraception within marriage as being morally responsible. I simply could not understand the Catholic position on this issue.

As I tried to come to grips intellectually with the church's teaching on contraception I found that many, if not most, of the arguments put forth in its defense were simply inadequate. This was true not only of the attempt of theologians to explain the issue, but even of authoritative papal documents. When Pius XI in *Casti Connubii* said that "any use of matrimony whatsoever in the exercise of which the act is deprived, by human interference of its natural power to procreate life, is an offense against the law of God and nature ...,"[5] he seemed to be trying to derive, illegitimately, an "ought" from an "is." In 1903, G.E. Moore effectively exposed the error of what he called this "naturalistic fallacy." One cannot determine what ought to be simply on the basis of what is, for, indeed, some things which *are* ought not to be. This naturalistic approach seemed to confuse the laws of nature with the moral law.

Another attempt to explain the immorality of contraception was the "perverted faculty" argument[6] which insisted that it was immoral to pervert a faculty by preventing it from fulfilling its proper function, in this case by preventing the genitalia from generating. However, persons often prevent faculties from performing their functions without any suggestion that doing so is immoral. The use of ear plugs is an obvious example which comes readily to mind.[7]

Although magisterial teaching does not derive its authority by how effectively it is presented, still, bad arguments have often rendered it less effective in motivating the faithful to conform their lives to the teaching. This is particularly true today in the industrialized nations with large educated populations. It was, in fact, not magisterial documents, but rather the philosophical and theological writings of Catholic lay scholars which finally were convincing to me and which made the magisterial position on contraception entirely intelligible and reasonable.[8]

As Professor Schüller has pointed out in his presentation, inadequate arguments have also been employed to explain magisterial teaching on some of the reproductive technologies discussed in the Instruction on Respect for Human Life in Its Origins and on the Diginity of Procreation. Some of the topics dealt with in the Instruction, such as homologous and heterologous artificial insemination, are not new to magisterial reflection. Some, such as in vitro fertilization and surrogate motherhood, are addressed for the first time in a formal manner.[9]

In his paper in this volume, Professor Schüller sees the declaration by Pius XII on the illicitness of artificial insemination as buttressed by naturalistic arguments which confuse the natural for the moral order. "It should not be overlooked," said the Pope, "that the conceiving of a new life according to the will and design of the Creator alone brings with it an astonishing degree of perfection in the actualizing of the intended goal." The effectiveness of the natural processes, however, cannot be used as a moral criterion for condemning artificial modes of reproduction. Professor Schüller presents a very thorough refutation of the naturalistic line of moral reasoning, and I find it convincing. He is, in my opinion, quite right when he states that the "difference ... between natural and artificial agency, purely in itself, never provides basis for making a moral judgment."

There have unfortunately been attempts in the Catholic tradition to make moral judgments on the basis of natural or artificial agency. This obviously does not reflect the best of our tradition but it seems always to have been there as a danger. It has sometimes even insinuated itself into the best of our tradition. We might wish that St. Thomas Aquinas had not incorporated Ulpian's definition of the natural law into his treatise on the law, but he did. Uplian had taught that the natural law was "that which nature has taught all animals."[10] That does not adequately express St. Thomas' own understanding of the natural law, but certain authors have subsequently fallen into the trap of confusing the laws of nature with the moral law. Certain established customs of the church only helped to reinforce this confusion. Forty years ago, for example, only natural fibers were to be used for sacred vestments and only candles of 100% beeswax could be burned in our churches. It was as though there was something immoral about the use of anything artificial such as synthetic fibers. This attitude was easily extended to the area of sexual conduct, where contraception was perceived as being immoral because it was artificial. This misunderstanding still persists today as people incorrectly refer to artificial contraception as being immoral and contrast it with natural contraception, which is deemed moral. The judgment, however, is incorrectly passed on the qualifier, not the act. It is contraception which is immoral, not the condition as to whether it is "artificially" or "naturally" practiced.

Again, there is sometimes confusion between the laws of nature and the natural law (a phrase I'm reluctant to use because of the misunderstanding it generates but which is unavoidable since it is so imbedded in the church's tradition). The laws of nature are descriptive while the natural law is prescriptive. The laws of nature describe what occurs time after time, while the natural law prescribes what ought to be done.

Every time a stone is released it falls to the ground. This occurs with such regularity that it appears that the stone is a conscious entity following a law, and so we speak metaphorically of a "law" of gravity which the stone "obeys." Of course, a stone is an inanimate object and, strictly speaking, rather than anthropomorphically speaking, obeys nothing.

The natural law is a moral law prescribing or directing human conduct. Here, "law" is used in a much more accurate way since a law is an ordinance of the reason and is applicable only to conscious, rational beings. As St. Thomas said, "Law is nothing else than an ordinance of reason for the common good, promulgated by him who has care of the community."[11]

The formulation and promulgation of laws is an activity natural to rational creatures whereby actions are ordered. The natural law is the human person's rational participation in the eternal law which itself orders all of creation.[12] It is nothing other than the human person ordering his own actions reasonably. The natural law is not a law of nature to which the human person passively conforms.[13] It, rather, is formulated by the person himself as he actively determines the goods on behalf of which he chooses to act. The rational creature, through the natural law, becomes "provident both for himself and for others," according to Aquinas.[14]

St. Thomas is aware of the distinction between the laws of nature, to which animals are subject, and the moral law formulated by the rational creature.

> Even irrational animals partake in their own way of the eternal reason, just as the rational creature does. But because the rational creature partakes thereof in an intellectual and rational manner, therefore the participation of the eternal law in the rational creature is *properly* called a law, since a law is something pertaining to reason ... Irrational creatures, however, do not partake thereof in a rational manner, and therefore there is no participation of the eternal law in them, *except by way of likeness.*[15]

So it is clear that St. Thomas himself does not fall prey to the confusing of the laws of nature with the moral law; of confusing the "is" with the "ought."

However, it is not morally irrelevant to take the "is" into consideration because the human person *is*, after all, rational. To act in accord with his nature does not mean to accept his lower animal nature as normative, but rather his higher rational nature.

The human person is most fully himself when acting reasonably because it is his rationality which most adequately and most faithfully characterizes him. How is it that we recognize when someone is acting in a most fully human, i.e., rational way? When one is seen as acting on behalf of ends perceived as goods, it is said that he is acting reasonably, humanly, morally. "Ends are to the practical intellect what principles are to the speculative."[16]

The end may occur last in terms of the execution of an act, but it is first in terms of the formulation of an act. As T.S. Eliot said, "The end is where we begin." The end is that on behalf of which we act and which makes a given act intelligible. It is said that a person is acting reasonably if the end on behalf of which, the purpose for which, he is acting can be perceived.

It is appropriate for humans, as rational creatures, to act on behalf of ends perceived as good, i.e., as things the possession of which will lead to happiness and a full flowering of one's humanity. Every person has a disposition toward fullness or wholeness, and one's natural inclinations provide clues as to what will constitute it. The goods humans naturally seek are "to be found only by examining all of man's basic tendencies. These prefigure everything man can achieve."[17] The inclinations are not animal drives to which we surrender, as an animal would to its instincts; but rather they point us toward those goods the possession of which generally adds to human happiness. The enumeration of the basic goods may vary but they are generally held to be life (in terms of the preservation of one's own life and of the species), knowledge, play, aesthetic experience, friendship and religion.[18] This is not an exhaustive list, of course, but does indicate the basic human goods on behalf of which we act.

One of the realities—and beauties—of life is that we are presented with more goods than we could ever hope to realize. One thing, however, which we ought not to do is to reject or act against any good as we choose to realize another, for to do so would undermine those very ends which make our actions intelligible. Indeed, it would be to act against or to undermine those very things which even make human conduct possible, for they constitute the ends on behalf of which we act, they present to us the possibilities of acting at all.

In this approach just outlined, it can be seen that the morality of an act is not determined in light of its conformity to some physical law of nature but rather of its conformity to or consonance with the reasonable nature of the acting person. The question of artificiality being a moral determinant is not even raised. Some of the language of magisterial documents to the contrary not withstanding, artificiality alone is not a morally determining factor. In fact, in an allocution in 1949 in which he declared homologous artificial insemination to be immoral, Pius XII stated, "Saying this does not necessarily proscribe the use of certain artificial means destined to facilitate the natural act ..."[19] And the Instruction under consideration here states quite explicitly and unequivocally, "These interventions [considered in the document] are not to be rejected on the grounds that they are artificial" (Intro. 3).

What primarily concerns one is not the literary genre or rhetorical devices used in the Instruction but rather the validity of its moral conclusions. What will be the moral determinants for the Instruction are certain values, meanings and goods "of the personal order," not the natural order. The very title of the document is instructive in this case: On Respect for Human Life in Its Origin and on the Dignity of Procreation. There are two fundamental human goods at stake which the magisterium, "inspired ... by the love which she owes to man" wishes to safeguard and promote: "the life of the human being called into existence and the special nature of the transmission of human life in marriage" (Intro. 4).

In all fairness to the authors of the document, it must be said that their sincere concern and solicitude for the human person in modern technological societies are obvious. There is no reason to think that the Instruction was issued for any other reason than in response to "requests for clarification and guidance" and out of "the love which [the church] owes to man" and a desire to advance only "the respect, defense and promotion of man" (Intro. 1). The approach of the Instruction is one of a reasoned exposition of basic human goods and values to be safeguarded and promoted. The document has on occasion been portrayed as being opposed to all "artificial" interventions, despite the disclaimer of the document itself and the fact that the authors specifically excluded passing a moral judgment on two current reproductive technologies, Lower Tubal Ovum Transfer (LTOT) and Gamete Intrafallopian Transfer (GIFT). Furthermore, the document was characterized as issuing prohibitions and condemnations in a harsh legal fashion. *The Washington Post* even called it a "Birth Edict." In all fairness, it must be pointed out that the document shows an admirable development within the Curia of moving away from legalistic language which regrettably did characterize many moral pronouncements in the past. Finally, it was widely reported that the church had declared artificial interventions to be mortal sins. It goes without saying that the term does not even appear in the document.

As indicated, through the Instruction the magisterium desires to protect and promote two basic human goods: the life of the human being called into existence and the special nature of the transmission of human life in marriage.

The first value at stake in the Instruction is human life itself, the very value primarily at stake in Paul VI's encyclical on the regulation of births, *Humanae Vitae*, "of human life." The concern of that encyclical was not artificial birth control, but rather the inestimable value of human life.

The dignity and value of the individual person is acknowledged in virtually every moral system, even in those which are agnostic or nontheistic. The founding documents of our nation declare that "all men are created equal and endowed by their Creator with certain inalienable rights: life, liberty, and the pursuit of happiness." Through his Categorical Imperative, Kant insisted that every person must be treated as an end in himself and can never be used as a means to an end. The inviolability of the human person is affirmed in such international and intercultural documents as the United Nations Declaration on the Rights of Man and the Helsinki Accords.

The human person is one of the goods on behalf of which we act and which makes contemplated actions intelligible. The flourishing of the person, for example, is the good which makes a surgeon's removal of a gangrenous leg moral and intelligible.

It is nothing other than the good of the human person which

is one of the objects of the Instruction, not some kind of impersonal biological process. The Instruction insists that it articulates a "moral teaching corresponding to the dignity of the human person." Its concern is that "the values and rights of the human person be safeguarded" (Intro. 5). Since it is concerned with life in its origin, the Instruction insists that "from the moment of conception, the life of every human being is to be respected in an absolute sense" (I1).

The second value which the Instruction seeks to safeguard is the dignity of procreation, i.e., "the special nature of the transmission of human life in marriage." Again, the discussion is of a human personal good, although this may not appear as self-evident as the other good. What constitutes the "dignity" of procreation? Again, it is in its ordering toward the good of human life. The dignity of procreation is seen in the acts appropriate to it being shared exclusively with only one other person, the spouse. The dignity of procreation is also seen in the fact that these acts take place only within marriage for the child's sake. Should the procreative good be realized through those acts which are apt for its realization it will require a stable, protective environment for its flourishing. It will require the family, an "environmental womb." Hence the dignity of procreation is acknowledged and safeguarded only within marriage, as the Instruction states.

But the document also speaks of the "special nature" of the transmission of life in marriage. This "special nature" is, quite bluntly, conjugal intercourse. Human life arises from, in the words of Canon Law, a "conjugal act which is per se suitable for the generation of children to which marriage is ordered by its nature and by which the spouses become one flesh."[20] In fact, the act which consummates a marriage and renders the bond forever indissoluble is a very, very human act; it is simply intercourse which the couple, in the words of the code, "have performed between themselves in a human manner."

The dignity of procreation is derived from our nature as *human* persons. We are psychosomatic realities. We live and move and have our being as bodies. We are indeed rational bodies, a formulation to be preferred to "embodied spirits," which seems to imply an accidental union of two disparate entities. We are our bodies. In its classical formulation it is said that "anima forma corporis est." We have no proper existence except as rational bodies and it is the "body that expresses the 'person'."[21] This is not a flaw; this is our perfection as human beings. When man first beheld woman he declared: "This is bone of my bones, and flesh of my flesh!" (Gn 2:23)

Yet there has always been a certain human uneasiness with this reality. Is it possible that the crown of creation should be subject to finitude, ignorance, passions, digestive processes, elimination of bodily waste, a less than tidy manner of reproduction? This dualistic temptation has always accompanied Christianity and has expressed itself in a multitude of ways; there have been the Gnostics and Manicheans and Bogomils and Cathari and Albigensians. Surely, they have insisted, we are better than this. This bodily untidiness does not truly reflect what we are. The loftier we are, the more we distance ourselves from these distasteful bodily functions.

With a little reflection it seems anyone of us could devise a better mode of reproduction ... one that was not so messy, so subject to frightfully unruly passions, so prone to misunderstanding and confusion and guilt.

There are indeed grave difficulties to being sexed realities, but it does constitute what we are—in our perfection. Despite all the problems, we are rational bodies, which means that we are sexed. Since we live and move and have our being as bodies, it is as bodies that we communicate with one another. It is the way by which we form that elemental community known as the family, and it is the way by which we perpetuate the species.

Now, to say that it would be preferable that we were not rational *animals*, but rather rational spirits, is not illogical or irrational, but it is in vain, since we cannot be other than we are; and it is unchristian, since we believe that the world as God created it, Creation as such, is good.

In the *Quaestiones Disputatae de Potentia Dei*, St. Thomas addresses the following argument: since God is incorporeal and our goal is to be like God, it must be that the soul separated from the body is more like God than the soul united with the body. Aquinas, in sound Christian fashion, replies boldly: "The soul united with the body is more like God than the soul separated from the body because it (the soul in the body) possesses its nature in a more complete fashion."[22]

Rather than rejecting the goodness of the body—as some critics of Catholicism claim—the church rather affirms it as the very means by which we glorify God. Ours is a very sensual religion. It was St. Paul who is usually accused of having an "antisex" attitude, and yet it is he who wrote: "Know you not that your bodies are members of Christ—Glorify and bear God in your bodies."[23] "And now, brothers, I beg you through the mercy of God to offer your bodies as a living sacrifice holy and acceptable to God, your spiritual worship."[24] "The wife has not power of her own body, but the husband. And in like manner, the husband also has not power of his own body, but the wife."[25] "In fact, husbands ought to love their wives as their own bodies."[26]

The way in which husband and wife express their love for one another is as human beings—through their bodies. Now obviously this is, to a certain degree, subject to the physical laws of nature. The laws of nature determine to a considerable degree the manner in which love and affection are expressed. As one author puts it, "Precisely because a slower and more gradual rise in the curve of sexual arousal is characteristic of the female organism the need for tenderness during physical intercourse, and also before it begins and after its conclusion, is explicable in purely biological terms. If we take into account the shorter and more violent curve of arousal in the man, an act of tenderness on his part in the context of marital intercourse requires the significance of an act of virtue ... specifically, the virtue of continence, and so indirectly the virtue of love."[27] The author of that advice was not Havelock Ellis or Dr. Ruth, but Karol Wojtyla, currently the Supreme Pontiff of the Catholic Church. Human sexual relations can never be reduced to the physical laws of nature, but they can also never be properly understood by ignoring these brute realities. This is true even when marriage is considered on the supernatural plane of sacrament. "Grace does not destroy nature, but presupposes and builds upon it."

All of this must be kept in mind when one considers the second value safeguarded in the Instruction: the dignity of procreation. An element of the dignity of procreation is this very physicality we have been discussing, those human acts which of themselves are apt for the generation of new life. We know that life can come into being by means other than an intimate personal act between a man and a woman. It has been done for generations with animals. However, as Pope John XXIII said, "The transmission of human *life* is entrusted by nature to a personal and conscious act ... For this reason one cannot use means and follow methods which could be licit in the transmission of the life of plants and animals."[28] Far from the transmission of human life being subjected to procedures and physical laws directing the transmission of animal life, human procreation is placed in the transcendent realm of human freedom and cocreation with God. The physicality of our sex is entirely informed by and imbued with our spiritual nature. As Cahal Daly writes, "Sex is never merely physical, biological; it expresses man's quest for absolutes, his desire for timeless happiness, for perfect mutual love and understanding, for unchanging lovableness, for unfailing faithfulness."[29] Such, however, can never be realized in our finite physical existence. Yet the physical love a man and woman have for one another draws them to such longings that neither can fulfill. In the words of Gustave Thibon, "Woman promises man what God alone can give."[30] And she promises this in and through her body.

In light of these reflections on the two basic goods promoted by the Instruction, human life and the dignity of procreation, what judgment is to be made of the various reproductive technologies mentioned in the Instruction? In order to see how they apply, a case will be chosen which is free of as many complicating moral issues as possible. This would be the case of homologous in vitro fertilization in which the gametes are provided by the spouses, the sperm is obtained by morally licit means (i.e., no masturbation), and only one ovum is fertilized so that there is no willful destruction of nascent life. It will also be assumed that there is no appreciable risk for the mother or the child in the procedures used.

In what way would the first value of respect for human life be treated by such a procedure? I do not believe it would show the respect due to the human person who is to be seen as autonomous, inviolable and of incomparable worth. As such, he is to be treated as an end in himself. Rather than the new life arising out of the human acts shared by the parents, it is manufactured out of the raw materials provided by husband and wife. The child is treated as an object, a thing manufactured out of an egg and sperm subject to quality control and domination by others. Such a manufacture of a person is inappropriate to his innate and unassailable worth. Such a procedure would subject human life to the arbitrary decisions of others and would constitute, in the words of the Instruction, a "dynamic of violence and domination" (II). "The one conceived must be the fruit of his parents' love. He cannot be desired or conceived as the product of an intervention of medical or biological techniques; that would be equivalent to reducing him to an object of scientific technology" (IIB4). To manufacture the child is to make him subordinate to his manufacturers. As William E. May says, "a human life, the life of a being that is the bearer of inviolable and inalienable rights, is not to be considered as a product inferior in nature and subordinate in value to its producers."[31] In an age which has witnessed the dreadful consequences of the objectification and subsequent abuse of the human person, the magisterium will speak out against any threat to the dignity of the individual person. This principle is so comprehensive that it will insist that even spouses who have married to create a family do not have "a true and proper 'right to a child'," so that they could use whatever means they chose to have the child.

Rather than advocating the Stoic adage that we ought to learn from the animals, the church insists that we do just the opposite, that we be fully human in our regard for the new life to be generated. In his book *Principles for a Catholic Morality*, Timothy O'Connell had written, "[the] fundamental ethical command imposed on the Christian is ... 'Be human'."[32] Pius XII had expressed the same truth differently: "To reduce the cohabitation of married persons and the conjugal act to a mere organic function for the transmission of the germs of life would be to convert the domestic hearth, sanctuary of the family, into nothing more than a biological laboratory."[33] In the procedures mentioned in the Instruction, the new life is manipulated into existence with the same degree of domination used to produce fruit flies or clone mice. As legitimate as the desire for a couple is to have children, they must recognize that no child is theirs by right—nor do they have the right to so dominate the child that they can bring it into being through any method they choose. In the child's unique and irrepeatable origin, in the words of the Instruction, "the child must be respected and recognized as equal in personal dignity to those who give him life" (IIB4). Instead, through homologous in vitro fertilization the child is manufactured to satisfy the desires of the parents. This is, in my opinion, a subjection of the child to the domination of technology, parents and technicians, and is not consonant with a child's innate worth and dignity. To use the imagery of William May, as the Word was eternally begotten of the Father, not made, even so the physical words of love spoken between spouses beget, they do not make, a new life of inestimable worth.[34] The human person is to be begotten, not made.

The other value to be threatened in homologous in vitro fertilization is the dignity of procreation. It was argued earlier that the totality of the marital act, its physical as well as its emotional and spiritual dimensions, the totality of the marital act is constitutive of its dignity. This ultimately points to the dignity of the persons, known as spouses, who engage in coitus. They are, in their perfection, rational bodies which are unavoidably sexed. It is in their perfection as rational bodies that they live and move and have their being. The only way in which they come to know reality and even God himself is in and through their bodies. The way in which they express their love for one another, forge an indissoluble bond between one another, and realize a new embodiment of their love in a child, is in and through their bodies. As the Instruction points out, "It is in their bodies and through their bodies that the spouses consummate their marriage and are able to become father and mother" (IIB4).

The *physicality* of conjugal coitus is part of the dignity of the act. Conception can take place without it—but it is a diminished act. Such a mode of conception is deprived of its human perfection; it is less than fully human and therefore beneath the dignity of a fully human act.

Furthermore, the acts ordered toward the procreation of new life are rightly conjugal acts, i.e., they are acts which are posited only by husband and wife out of recognition of the exclusivity of their love for one another and of the uniqueness of the relationship which will provide the environmental womb (the family) for their child. However, with homologous in vitro fertilization it is obvious that the child has not been engendered by the mutual coital expression of love of the couple, but has been manufactured by a third party or parties, by the physician and biological technicians. It is the physician who is manufacturing the child, and this intrusion deprives procreation of its dignity which it has only when it is conjugal, that is, realized physically between a husband and wife in a life-long, exclusive relationship. Rather than arising out of the exclusive, sexual expressions of love of his parents, the child is manufactured through a joint-venture agreement entered into by his parents and a third party.

These acts of control, domination and manipulation associated with reproductive technologies are fraught with danger for the child and for the adults involved. It has already led to the destruction of and experimentation with nascent life, and the sad drama of Baby M.

We are truly free and fully human only when we act on behalf of goods, in this case, human life and the dignity of procreation, and do nothing to assault or diminish these goods which provide the intelligibility of our sexual actions and make them possible.

Notes

1. Second Vatican Council, *Lumen Gentium*, in Walter Abbott, ed., *Documents of Vatican II* (New York: Guild Press, 1966), 25.

2. Ibid, 21.

3. C. Henry Peschke, *Christian Ethics*, vol. 2 (Dublin: C. Goodliffe Neale, 1978), 42-43.

4. For example, see John C. Ford, S.J., and Gerald Kelly, S.J., "Doctrinal Value and Interpretation of Papal Teaching" in *Readings in Moral Theology, No. 3: The Magisterium and Morality* (New York: Paulist Press, 1982).

5. Pius XI, *Casti Connubii* (December 31, 1930).

6. Henry Davis, S.J., "Birth Control: The Perverted Faculty Argument," *Ecclesiastical Review* 81 (1929): 54-69.

7. Germain Grisez, *Contraception and Natural Law* (Milwaukee: The Bruce Publishing Co., 1964), 27ff. for an effective refutation of the perverted faculty argument.

8. Grisez, *Contraception*; John Finnis, *Natural Law and Natural Rights* (Oxford: Clarendon Press, 1980).

9. In vitro fertilization was alluded to cursorily and rejected out of hand by Pius XII in his address to members of the Second World Congress on Fertility and Sterility, 16 May 1954.

10. St. Thomas Aquinas, *Summa Theologica* (New York: McGraw Hill/Blackfriars, 1964), 1a2ae, 94. 2.

11. Ibid., 1a2ae, 90, 4.

12. Ibid., 1a2ae, 91, 2.

13. Ibid.

14. Ibid.

15. Ibid., 1a2ae, 91, 2, 3.

16. Ibid., 1a2ae, 65, 1.

17. Grisez, *Contraception*, 63.

18. John Finnis, *Natural Law and Natural Rights* (Oxford: Clarendon Press, 1980), 85-95.

19. Pius XII, "Medical Ethics," Allocution to the International Congress of Catholic Doctors, 29 September 1949, *Catholic Mind* 48 (1950):250-53.

20. Code of Canon Law, Canon 1061.

21. John Paul II, *Original Unity of Man and Woman: Catechists on the Book of Genesis* (Boston: St. Paul Editions, 1981), 109.

22. St. Thomas Aquinas, *Questiones Disputatae de Potentia Dei*, 5, 10, ad 5.

23. 1 Cor 6:15, 20.

24. Rom 12:1.

25. 1 Cor 7:4.

26. Eph 5:28.

27. Karol Wojtyla, *Love and Responsibility* (New York: Farrar, Straus and Giroux, 1981), 275.

28. John XXIII, *Mater et Magistra*, quoted in the Instruction, Introduction, 4.

29. Cathal B. Daly, *Morals, Law and Life* (Chicago: Scepter, 1966), 43.

30. Gustave Thibon, *What God Has Joined Together* (London: Hollis & Carter, 1952), 178.

31. William E. May, "Begotten, Not Made," *Perspectives in Bioethics* (Cromwell, Conn: Pope John Paul II Bioethics Center, 1983), 54.

32. Timothy O'Connell, *Principles for a Catholic Morality* (New York: The Seabury Press, 1978), 40.

33. Pius XII, "Medical Ethics," 29 September 1949.

34. May, "Begotten, Not Made," 54.

Elio Sgreccia

Moral Theology and Artificial Procreation in Light of Donum Vitae*

I. Introduction

Our task, in this report, is to emphasize and, if possible, to obtain a thorough knowledge of the reasons, or moral-theological motivations, that inspire the practical implications and responses of the Instruction of the Congregation for the Doctrine of the Faith on Respect for Human Life in its Origin and on the Dignity of Procreation. Our task is to pursue a study of hermeneutics that could help us to understand better such practical implications and the range of values to which they belong. This task, which we can only indicate here, will need further contributions and elaboration.

As an introduction I would like, first of all, to make a triple preliminary statement on: (a) the cultural context in which the new methods of artificial human procreation—those to which we refer by the term "procreative"—rise and establish themselves; (b) the limits of biotechnology when it is applied to the human person; (c) the role of the magisterium and its value in this field. After these preliminary statements I shall continue by emphasizing the major points of moral theology which are expressed or implied in the Instruction. In concluding, I shall suggest some methods which, in my opinion, should stimulate further ethical and theological reflection.

* Translated by Cristina Demagistris, L'Université de Genève, L'Ecole de Traduction et d'Interpretation.

A. The Cultural Context

Both the technologies applied to the procedures of procreation, and those more properly defined as genetic engineering of the human person, are part of a broad undertaking of inestimable importance that could be defined as the project of "anthropotechnics." Western man, after coming to understand the mystery of the atom and overcoming the barriers of the force of earth's gravity through space travel, can now dominate the procedures of human procreation and can also manipulate the genetic identity of the human individual. We are talking about the greatest and most Promethean project ever expressed in the history of culture and science.

This project questions the relationship between love and life within procreation, between person and nature within the individual, between freedom and responsibility toward future generations, between ethics and technique within human behavior. We can think of the affirmation of C.S. Lewis, who observes, "When we will be free to do whatever we want to with our species ... then we will have won the battle ... But who will have won it precisely? In fact, the power of man to do with himself whatever he pleases means ... the power of some men to do what they want with other men." The masters of the human species will be those called by Lewis the "conditioners."[1]

This event and its possibility cannot be underestimated. When Oppenheimer worked on the construction of the atom bomb, he is said to have declared, "We are working for the devil."[2]

Today we hope that all those who thought that atomic instruments would be a useful means to avoid wars are now persuaded, or will be soon, that the best guarantee against the use of atomic weapons is their disassembly if they have already been built, or the discontinuance of all construction of such weapons.

It would have been better, in Oppenheimer's time, to discuss the ethical limits of atomic research and experimentation in order to direct researchers exclusively to pacific uses, and to avoid financial waste and human sacrifice.

I believe we should keep in mind three factors that, in my opinion, constitute the crux of the matter and represent three risks or dangers of human and cultural catastrophe at this point in human history. These factors must be made known in order to understand fully the prophetic value of the Congregation's document. The first factor is the attempt to *destroy* the concept of the human person; the second is the attempt to *dominate and control* the procedures of procreation and of procreated life; the third is the very obvious attempt to establish a *utilitarian ethic,* or social consent, and with this ethic, the destruction of any objective consistency of ethical values and norms. The profound value of the Instruction and its prophetic meaning is to be found in the rejection of these three attempts.

The Destruction of the Concept of the Person. To be sure, it is difficult to sketch an accurate description of the human person, because it is a larger reality than the name and concept themselves. But it is a fact that the reality "hypostasis," as the Greeks called it, or "person," according to the Latin thinkers' appellation, is intended to signify the absolute newness represented by the individual human being compared to the rest of the universe. The person *transcends* the universe and, because of the spirit that characterizes it, marks the opening to eternity. Today the term "person" is no longer being used as a transcendent boundary between the human and the nonhuman universe, but is being used in a *discriminatory* way, that is, within the human universe, between two phases of its development, on the basis of merely biological, psychological or sociological criteria. A person would be the born child, or maybe the fetus, but not the embryo. In some opinions, the malformed child that does not have a high quality of life, or the dying individual who loses consciousness, is no longer a person. The person is not considered as such for what *he or she is,* but for what he or she can do or what he or she appears to be.

This is the first and worst *discrimination* among human beings and within the human being himself: in short, "I" would be the same"I" now, at thirty, forty or fifty, compared to what I was at the age of three months or three days. Who decides, and on what basis is this ontological distinction made? According to those who make this discrimination, some human beings would be persons whereas others would not; and these same individuals would be persons when others want to recognize them as such, and not when they begin to exist as unique individuals who cannot be duplicated.

The second attempt to destroy the concept of the person is *control over the procedures of procreation*. This began with contraception and now continues, in a more serious way, with artificial procreation.

The contraceptive incentive was justified by the problems couples had concerning birth control. But it soon became a *political methodology* and a strategy of colonization for the most developed and influential countries to affect the demographic development of emerging peoples. Contraception has become a means of demographic control through linking economic aid to the obligation of family planning. Perhaps a "White Paper" should appear in order to expose and denounce the degree to which contraception, abortion, and sterilization have been imposed on the world by well-identified economic forces and international organizations, hankering for control.

The pill has become a political weapon and a means of economic power, Very few—too few—people thanked the church and, in particular, Paul VI who, in *Humanae Vitae*, declared that life and conjugal love are indivisible, and that man has no power over them. What was considered by the press as a document contrary to the freedom of women was actually a strong and solitary defense of procreative freedom.

Procreation within conjugal union, respecting the totality of the person, according to a plan of love and shared responsibility: this was and is the essential point for safeguarding procreative freedom.[3] With artificial procreation a further step is taken, because control is no longer imposed within the sexual act, but outside it, so that the beginning of human life appears as the result of an external causality, extrinsic and different from the conjugal act. The biologist makes the embryo and keeps control over it. Procreation is not closely related to the *act* of conjugal love, but to the biologist's *technical activity*.

The Congregation's Instruction stresses that extracorporal procreation is not respectful of the dignity of either the spouses or the future child, or the conjugal character of marriage. It "entrusts the life and identity of the embryo into the power of doctors and biologists and establishes the domination of technology over the origin and destiny of the human person. Such a relationship of domination is itself contrary to the dignity and equality that must be common to parents and children" (IIB5).

Tryanny, deplored in the political world, is transferred to the biological world, and once it is there, it is impossible to drive it away. The art of the possible, which was considered as the law that regulated politics, becomes the norm of biology and is transformed into the art of biotechnological power. We are all aware of the fact that experimentation, checks and changes are made on the embryo in vitro just as on any other laboratory product. Who will be able to prevent this power from expanding and being planned in the world? The procreative act is not something that the married couple can transfer to the biologists, the doctors, or the state.

The third development taking place before us, and as a justification of the two previous ones, is the *introduction of ethical utilitarianism*, to justify the intervention into procreation and the family. Neither the anthropology of the person nor that of nature is accepted; they are both considered fixed and medieval. What is right and what is not should depend on "social consent," "social utility" or intentions. Is no one wondering what would be the terms of comparison or who would be the arbiter of these consents and utilities?

Today utilitarian ethics is fierce and employs many strategies: social utility, evolution of customs and values, proportionalism, and so forth. These theories are very sophisticated, so that a careful analysis is required to expose their pseudo-justifications. All relativist and utilitarian ethics contain the following point: utility is defined by those who can define it, those who have the power to manage consents, to estimate the worth of men and decide their usefulness and destination.

Thus the embryo would not be defined for what it is, but for what it can be considered; the quality of the life of the future child, which is necessary in order to have the right to be born, would be decided by those who are already adult, on the basis of the results of their diagnosis, of an "even distribution" of values, social expenses, and so forth.

The Instruction, emphasizing the inestimable value of the person, and directing consciences to the defense of human life in its origins, is offering safety and safeguard not only to human beings undergoing elimination in their embryonic stage, but also to ethics in its objective values that respect the totality of human life.

B. The Limits of Technology

It is neither necessary nor possible here to stress the positive aspects of technological progress, especially the progress of the last fifty years, for the benefit of human knowledge and of medicine itself. Technology does not have to be evaluated only in relation to the object that it produces and transforms, but also in relation to the subject that creates technology, that is, the human person. In this way, all technological means, or technology itself, can be considered as a new kind of experimental science, and it can be seen, especially in its application phase, as the expansion of human *corporeity*. As technology has progressed, the human body has broadened and developed in its muscular and mechanical capacity, in its sensory capacity (today we can "see" a man anywhere in the world, even when he is landing on the moon), and now we can enhance neuronic capacities and mental skills up to a selective calculus through computer science and through what is called "artificial intelligence." But, according to the scientists, even those who adhere to neopositivist philosophy, technological development implies three serious risks that must be avoided.

Above all is its destructive power which, because of the perfection of technology itself, is defined as "catastrophic"[4] every time the risk is not contained. With technological progress today, no risks can be taken; on the contrary, risk has to be reduced to zero. This is valid for atomic energy and also, in my opinion, for genetic engineering and the manipulation of human procreation.

Second, with regard to the human subject, technology inevitably implies a "reduction" of human totality. Technology can only express what can be "reduced" to a measurable and unrepeatable quantity: it cannot be the *"source and spring"* of creativity and spirituality: it can copy a poem, but it cannot create a work of art.

The third and most serious danger is that of leading man to a state of dependency upon technology, so that he will feel inferior to his products that, in terms of material strength, surpass and influence him. This is the situation that makes man see even himself as a "technical" object, a robot—the situation that has been called "Promethean shame."[5] C.S. Lewis, a philosopher of neopositivist background, writes, "The real objection is that if man chooses to treat himself as raw material, material he will be."[6] And also, "Every new power attained by man is also power over man ... the final stage will take place when man, through eugenics, influence before birth, instruction and propaganda based on perfect applied psychology, will have acquired full control of himself."[7] A rigid control of the few over the many and over the entire personality makes the subjectivity of the many treatable as an object.

This is why, as the Pope said, "Scientific progress cannot be set on a neutral ground. The ethical norm, based on respect for the dignity of the person, has to enlighten and regulate both the phase of research and that of the application of its results."[8] In order to prevent man from becoming an object and product of technology, a global ethical growth of mankind is necessary, as well as a clear and broad vision of ethical orientation, plus a perception of the limits beyond which the subject-man can become the slave of his own technology.

The Instruction, which is the object of our study, maintains that "science and technology require, for their own intrinsic meaning, an unconditional respect for the fundamental criteria of the moral law: that is to say, they must be at the service of the human person, of his inalienable rights, and his true and integral good according to the design and will of God"[9] (Intro. 2).

C. Role and Value of the Magisterium

I intentionally spent a significant amount of time characterizing the cultural context to which the recent discoveries and applications of artificial procreation belong. In this way, the responsibility, role and value of the magisterium in this field will emerge more clearly.

In its conclusion the text of the Instruction affirms:

In particular, the Congregation for the Doctrine of the Faith addresses an invitation with confidence and encouragement to theologians, and above all to moralists, that they study more deeply and make ever more accessible to the faithful the contents of the teaching of the church's magisterium in the light of a valid anthropology in the matter of sexuality and marriage and in the context of the necessary interdisciplinary approach. Thus they will make it possible to understand ever more clearly the reasons for and the validity of this teaching. By defending man against the excesses of his own power, the church of God reminds him of the reasons for his true nobility; only in this way can the possibility of living and loving with that dignity and liberty which derive from respect for the truth be insured for the men and women of tomorrow. The precise indications which are offered in the present Instruction therefore are not meant to halt the effort of reflection, but rather to give it a renewed impulse in unrenounceable fidelity to the teaching of the church.

It is clearly stated in this passage that the church, together with its magisterium, is willing to help contemporary man to protect himself against "the excesses of his own power," and is aware of the fact that it has to insure to the men and women of tomorrow the possibility of living and loving, in respect for dignity, liberty and truth. At the same time, this passage reminds us of the double task of the moralist: investigate more deeply the reasons given by the magisterium to support the ethical indications, and make the teaching accessible to the faithful. Therefore, it is not a matter of further discussing the indications and evaluations offered by the magisterium, but rather of investigating their reasons. Also, it is not a matter of simply "taking note" of this teaching with "silent deference," but of making it *accessible* to our contemporaries through a positive effort of mediation.

The magisterium's competence in this field cannot first be questioned simply because we are dealing with issues related to biology and medicine. In fact, the Instruction does not intend to give its opinion about scientific matters, but about the biotechnological applications that are used in relation to human procreation and life in its origins. The very object of the teaching is the dignity of procreation and the defense of human life. In its introduction, the Instruction affirms:

> The church's magisterium does not intervene on the basis of a particular competence in the area of the experimental sciences; but having taken account of the data of research and technology, it intends to put forward, by virtue of its evangelical mission and apostolic duty, the moral teaching corresponding to the dignity of the person and to his or her integral vocation. It intends to do so by expounding the criteria of moral judgment as regards the application of scientific research and technology, especially in relation to human life and its beginnings. These criteria are the respect, defense and promotion of man, his "primary and fundamental right" to life, his dignity as a person who is endowed with a spiritual soul and with moral responsibility and who is called to beatific communion with God.

The Instruction refers to its own "evangelical mission and apostolic duty"; it refers to the fundamental and primary values of man, such as the dignity of the person, the fundamental value of life, and the dignity of procreation; it requests the specific reception that the church's magisterium deserves.

We are not simply confronting an "authoritative" opinion, but the voice of the magisterium and the practice of the doctrinal and pastoral duty of the church. We are not facing a simple and temporary point of view. The document, therefore, is an incentive for investigation and an unquestionable datum for theological and moral research.

Moreover, this teaching concludes a series of indications of the papal magisterium that already define many of the issues the Instruction deals with: the condemnation of abortion and the dignity of the embryo to be respected as a human person from the very moment of conception;[10] the indivisibility of the unitive dimension and of the conjugal act, and the consequent condemnation of heterologous insemination.[11] Numerous theologians thought these indications would be enough for an evaluation of artificial procreation considered in itself,[12] whereas other theologians believed that these indications would not be enough for a final judgment of homologous artificial procreation (IA homologous and FIVET homologous).[13]

The Instruction, confirming some of the issues already defined in previous pronouncements, also offers an unequivocal answer to the uncertain issues. Such an answer is coherent and consistent with the position of the magisterium.

This aspect of continuity, this normative qualification expressed by the words of the Instruction, the importance of the problems examined both in regard to themselves and compared to contemporary cultural trends—all of these lead to the conclusion that this document (the Instruction) has to be received by theologians and the faithful with the religious respect deserved by the church's magisterium. And we must recognize in it the sapiential gift of the Spirit with which "man can, in faith, contemplate and enjoy the mystery of God's plan."[14] There is no need to emphasize that it is the duty of the church's magisterium to "interpret authentically the word of the Lord, written or conveyed,"[15] and also the problems that arise from the interpretation of the word of the Lord that is printed and engraved in creation and in human creatures.

Paul VI recalled precisely this fact in *Humanae Vitae*:

> No member of the faithful could possibly deny that the church is competent in her magisterium to interpret the natural moral law. It is in fact indisputable, as Our predecessors have many times declared, that Jesus Christ, when He communicated His divine power to Peter and the other Apostles and sent them to teach all nations His commandments, constituted them as the authentic guardians and interpreters of the whole moral law, not only, that is, of the law of the Gospel but also of the natural law. For the natural law, too, declares the will of God, and its faithful observance is necessary for men's eternal salvation.[16]

It is true that today many faithful, often influenced by subjectivism in ethical deliberation and by utilitarianism in research, find it difficult to accept the magisterium's indications as a gift of truth and as a contribution to knowledge. This is why theology will have to work assiduously on rational penetration, enlightenment and dialogue in order to further the objective and complete consideration of this teaching. Theology must do this by developing, in particular, the implicit meaning and values of a richer humanism that includes the doctrine of the Instruction, and by presenting the ethical indications as a safeguard for the truth and liberty of the human person.

With this double attention to the indications of the Instruction and today's culture, I wish to suggest a few elements and focal points of a moral-theological character from which I think it is possible to define the terms of a positive dialogue.

Significant Points of the Instruction. The Instruction itself indicates "the fundamental values connected with the techniques of artificial procreation" and affirms that there are two: "the life of the human being called into existence and the special nature of the transmission of human life in marriage," adding that "the moral judgment on such methods of artificial procreation must therefore be formulated in reference to these values" (Intro. 4).

I think that, in order to clarify the connection between the two and, at the same time, open the dialogue more easily with contemporary culture, it is necessary to add a third intermediate value between the value of life and the value of procreation; this is the value of human corporeity. Cardinal Ratzinger himself, during the press conference for the presentation of the Instruction, mentioned this value of corporeity as one of the fundamental keys for reading the document. It is obvious that all of these values—life, corporeity, and procreation—are to be considered in the light of creation and of the personalistic conception of man.

A. Creation: Human Life as a Gift of Love in Love

The Holy Father told the participants at the Congress of the Catholic Association of Health Officers (ACOS): "It is clear that a culture established on the basis of man as master of man makes any foundation of human rights weak and unstable. And should such a culture become dominant, the future of mankind would be seriously threatened." And he added,

Unfortunately, signs of such a future are already visible in legalized abortion, euthanasia, in vitro insemination, physical violence considered as a legitimate means of struggle. This indicates how urgent it is to repropose the values of Christian culture, which affirms that man is a creation created and wanted by God; that God and not man is the source and measure of good; that a moral order which transcends man exists.[17]

This speech of the Holy Father views in vitro insemination as a sign of man's domination over man, which is contrary to respect for life considered as God's gift and a transcendent value. "In this hypothesis," the Holy Father said in the same speech, "the human being no longer has an absolute meaning and an inviolable value in himself; so he becomes as all other things, a manipulable instrument of production and consumption."[18]

In order to understand this major point more clearly, we must quote and compare two passages of the Instruction: the first is part of the introduction and the second is in the second part, where the evaluation of homologous artificial procreation is treated. In the introduction, the fact of creation by God and the fact of procreation according God's design are linked.

From the moment of conception, the life of every human being is to be respected in an absolute way because man is the only creature on earth that God has "wished for himself" and the spiritual soul of each man is immediately created by God: his whole being bears the image of the Creator. Human life is sacred because from its beginning it involves "the creative action of God" and it remains forever in a special relationship with the Creator, who is its sole end. God alone is the Lord of life from its beginning until its end: no one can, in any circumstance, claim for himself the right to destroy directly an innocent human being.

Human procreation requires on the part of the spouses responsible collaboration with the fruitful love of God; the gift of human life must be actualized in marriage through the specific and exclusive acts of husband and wife, in accordance with the laws inscribed in their persons and in their union[19] (Intro. 5).

The difference is therefore between life as a *gift* and life as a *product*.

In its second part, the Instruction says:

> The human person must be accepted in his parents' act of union and love; the generation of a child must therefore be the fruit of that mutual giving which is realized in the conjugal act wherein the spouses cooperate as servants and not as masters in the work of the Creator who is Love.
>
> In reality, the origin of a human person is the result of an act of giving. The one conceived must be the fruit of his parents' love. He cannot be desired or conceived as the product of an intervention of medical or biological techniques; that would be equivalent to reducing him to an object of scientific technology. No one may subject the coming of a child into the world to conditions of technical efficiency which are to be evaluated according to standards of control and dominion (IIB4).

That this link of creation-procreation can be maintained within God's design only if actualized through spousal union and the conjugal act, indicates not only the obligation of respect for the life of the conceived human being (and the consequent duty of avoiding abortion, nontherapeutic experimentation, physical damage to the embryo—moral norms that can also be derived from simple medical deontology), but also characterizes *how* the creature can be legitimately conceived.

Contemporary culture, which is sensitive to the value of liberty and yet has not been entirely victorious in giving anyone the guarantee to be born and develop in the name of liberty, will find a valuable contribution to the civilization of man in the church's message. *Only if conception is the fruit of human love and not of deterministic technique, will the human being enter history supported by love and free from biotechnological influence.*

The objections which are raised concerning this point are well known: even in homologous artificial insemination spousal love plays its role, since the spouses wish the coming of the new life. But we also know that this *intentionality* or subjective will is not enough to establish integrally the morality of the procreative act. As a matter of fact, it does not rescue the new human being from the technical domination exercised by biologists, and from all the consequences that could possibly stem from this fact.

According to the Instruction,

> Homologous IVF and ET is brought about outside the bodies of the couple through actions of third parties whose competence and technical activity determine the success of the procedure. Such fertilization entrusts the life and identity of the embryo to the power of doctors and biologists and establishes the domination of technology over the origin and destiny of the human person. Such a relationship of domination is in itself contrary to the dignity and equality that must be common to parents and children. (IIB5)[20]

From a theological point of view, therefore, artificial procreation presents itself as a severing of the link of obedience between procreators and creator; it implies the refusal of God's transcendent design; and it implies a secular relapse—beyond the subjects' intentions—into an attempt at immanent government and domination of procreation.

From an anthropological point of view, artificial procreation establishes a relationship of *domination of man over man* in his coming into life and in his first moment of existence in the world.

B. The Human Person and His Body

Another fundamental point which deserves further thought and development, rich in both theological and cultural suggestions, is to be found in the concept of corporeity, which is recalled in the Instruction and is characteristic of Christian anthropology. We cannot examine here the theories that many contemporary philosophical schools—from phenomenology to existentialism and structuralism—have developed concerning the value of the body. Nor can we give proper attention to the work of the Holy Father concerning the connection between corporeity and person, and between corporeity and sexuality.[21]

First, the human body, considered as individualized *physical life*, is defined, according to the previous magisterium, as a "fundamental value" of the person, in the embryonic stage from the first instance in which this corporeity becomes a human being, that is, from the moment of fertilization.

> Physical life, with which the course of human life begins, certainly does not itself contain the whole of a person's value, nor does it represent the supreme good of man who is called to eternal life. However, it does constitute in a certain way the "fundamental" value of life, precisely because upon this physical life all the other values of the person are based and developed. The inviolability of the innocent human being's right to life from the moment of conception until death is a sign and requirement of the very inviolability of the person to whom the Creator has given the gift of life (Intro. 5).

This statement qualifies the body as the "incarnation" of the person, and gives concrete and rational realism to the church's whole oral doctrine on the defense of human life in its origins, leaving out of consideration the different definitions given by various humanistic disciplines, and clarifying the medieval dispute about the moment of animation.

Corporeity is also considered as an *organic unity* of parts that have a meaning in relation to the entire organism and the entire person. From this point of view, corporeity *establishes* and clarifies the principle of totality, or therapeutic principle, which is also recalled by the Instruction concerning interventions into the human embryo.

Before treating the various questions concerning intervention into the human embryo and procreation, the Instruction begins with the following question:

> What moral criteria must be applied in order to clarify the problems posed today in the field of biomedicine? The answer to this question presupposes a proper idea of the nature of the human person in his bodily dimension.

For it is only in keeping with his true nature that the human person can achieve self-realization as a "unified totality," and this nature is, at the same time, corporal and spiritual. By virtue of its substantial union with a spiritual soul, the human body cannot be considered as a mere complex of tissues, organs and functions, nor can it be evaluated in the same way as the body of animals; rather, it is a constitutive part of the person who manifests and expresses himself through it (I2-4).

The "natural moral law," the Instruction continues, "expresses and lays down the purposes, rights and duties which are based upon the corporal and spiritual nature of the human person. Therefore, this law cannot be thought of as simply a set of norms on the biological level: rather, it must be defined as the rational order whereby man is called by the Creator to direct and regulate his life and actions and, in particular, to make use of his own body (Intro. 3).

But corporeity is understood by the Instruction and unanimously by the most recent biological and philosophical sciences, as *manifestation, epiphany, language of the person*, particularly with regard to sexuality in the male-female relationship.

As far as artificial procreation is concerned, the Instruction specifies that artificial procreation, since it is done through a technical act, corrodes the unity of the human being and the unity of body and spirit.

The moral value of the intimate link between the goods of marriage and between the meanings of the conjugal act is based upon the unity of the human being, a unity involving body and spiritual soul. Spouses mutually express their personal love in "body language," which clearly involves both "spousal meanings" and parental ones (IIB4b).

It is not difficult to understand that the bodily and spiritual unity of the spouses is violated when heterologous procreative techniques are used: in these cases (AI heterologous, IVF and ET heterologous) the unity of marriage is violated through recourse to donors (and also through recourse to surrogate motherhood). It is necessary, however, to understand the need for this corporal and spiritual union also within the conjugal act between the spouses.

C. The Conjugal Act: Its Unity and Plenitude

The third major moral point, which qualifies the Instruction and still causes quite a few problems, is the relationship involved in procreation—that between the human body and the conjugal act. This point is related to homologous artificial procreation and, in particular, to the prospect of a homologous human procreative procedure that could be free from any connection to other illicit acts (dispersion of embryos, surplus of embryos, masturbation to obtain the seed). Within the Catholic community it is relatively easy to understand rationally the condemnation of artificial procreative technologies every time they imply the interruption of human life in its origins or the donation of gametes. There has been significant argumentation of the hypothesis of the so-called *"simple case,"* which is still difficult to understand.

I think it is on this precise point that the Instruction better clarifies the human and theological plenitude of the procreative act. According to the Instruction,

> The conjugal act by which the couple mutually express their self-gift at the same time expresses openness to the gift of life. It is an act which is inseparably corporal and spiritual. It is in their bodies and through their bodies that the spouses consummate their marriage and are able to become father and mother. In order to respect the language of their bodies and their natural generosity, the conjugal union must take place with respect for its openness to procreation; and the procreation of a person must be the fruit and the result of married love. The origin of the human being thus follows from a procreation that is "linked to the union, not only biological but also spiritual, of the parents, made one by the bond of marriage." Fertilization achieved outside the bodies of the couple remains by this very fact deprived of the meanings and values which are expressed in the language of the body and in the union of human persons (IIB4b).

An act of procreation without bodily expression deprives this act not of the biological factor (which can be recovered technologically through the transfer of gametes), but rather of the personal communion that can be expressed only through the body in its plenitude and unity. The characteristic of spousal love is, as we know, the totality of the gift of the two persons. The substitution of the bodily act with technology is a "reduction" of the conjugal act; it means that the conjugal act is degraded to the typology of technical acts. Here again we encounter the intrinsic "reduction" which is characteristic of technology.

The technical act which *builds the object* is something else; the object remains ontologically nonhomogeneous compared to the subject; and the subject who built the object can dominate it. Similarly, the act which *expresses the subject* to another subject, whose equality he respects and with whom free expression and communion are allowed, is another thing. Among the expressive acts or languages of the body, the conjugal act is the one that has the characteristic of *plenitude* and *totality*: to reduce procreation to a technological fact, therefore, means to establish a relationship of domination, "producer subject—produced object"; it also means to degrade and impoverish the procreative act from both a theological and an anthropological point of view. In relation to the conjugal act, here again is affirmed the necessity of that unity and totality required by the whole spousal union: what is valid for marriage and conjugal life is also valid for the individual acts that express and realize it.

This vision, which refers to plenitude and totality, does not deserve the accusations of strictness or rigidity that some people find in the Instruction and in the teaching of the church. Conception accomplished without affection but by simple instinct would not be human. In the same way, a procreative act devoid of full personal and bodily communion would not be completely human.

Conclusion

I think that the task of theologians is to urge scientists and doctors to continue their research, as the Instruction affirms, in order to improve and offer those techniques that could serve as *simple aids* to conception and to the completion of conjugal effort. In addition, scientists and doctors should study new methods for prevention and authentic therapy of infertility (IIB6).

I think that what appears as "prohibition" today can turn into "prophecy" tomorrow. I also think that reflection upon the Instruction can be an incentive for everyone to rediscover and reaffirm the full humanism (all the human values in every person) that is threatened by the technological myth and by the excesses of technology applied to man without respect for the "human."

Notes

1. C.S. Lewis, *The Abolition of Man* (Milan: Jaca Book, 1979), 62-63; M. Paolinelli, "Natura Umana e Persona Umana: La Dignità della Procreazione," in E. Sgreccia, ed., *Il Dono della Vita* (Milan: Vita e Pensiero, 1987), 80.

2. V. Sidel, "Warfare," in W.T. Reich, ed., *Encyclopedia of Bioethics* (New York: Macmillan and Free Press, 1982).

3. E. de LaGrange et al., *Il Complotto Contro La Vita* (Milan: Ares, 1987); A. Fonseca, "Politische, Demografische e Contraccezione Oggi nel Mondo," *Civiltà Cattòlica* 3200 (1983): 134-48; E. Tremblay, *L'Affaire Rockefeller: L'Europe Occidentale en Danger* (Malmaison: Reul, 1979).

4. P. Lagadec, *La Civilisation du Risque* (Paris: Seuil, 1981).

5. A. Bausola, *Prolusione al 57^ Corso di Aggiornamento su Technologia ed Etica* (Milan: Vita e Pensiero); Paolinelli, "Natura Umana," 74ff.

6. Lewis, *Abolition of Man*, 63.

7. Ibid., 70-75; Bausola, *Prolusione*.

8. John Paul II, "The Person Is the Measure of Everything Human," 27 October 1980, *Origins* 10 (1980):351-52.

9. See also, Second Vatican Council, *Gaudium et Spes*, in Walter Abbott, ed., *The Documents of Vatican II* (New York: Guild Press, 1966), 35.

10. Pius XII, "The Duty of Physicians," 12 November 1944, in *The Pope Speaks* (New York: Pantheon Books, 1957), 109-17; Pius XII, "The Dignity of the Human Body," 21 May 1948, *The Catholic Mind* 46 (1948):488-92; Pius XII, "Apostolate of the Midwife," 29 October 1951, in V. Yzermans, *The Unwearied Advocate: Public Addresses of Pius XII* (St. Cloud, Minn.: St. Cloud Bookshop, 1956), 117-32; Pius XII, "Morality in Marriage," 27 November 1951, in Yzermans, 132-36; *Gaudium et Spes*, nos. 27 and 51; Paul VI, *Humanae Vitae*, 25 July 1968 (New York: Paulist Press, 1968); Paul VI, "Defense of the Right to Birth," 9 December 1972, in *The Teachings of Paul VI* (Washington, D.C.: U.S. Catholic Conference, 1973), 320-23; Paul VI, "On Human Conception," 7 September 1974, in *The Teachings of Paul VI*, 323-25; John Paul II, *Familiaris Consortio*, 22 November 1980, *Origins* 11(1981):437-66; John Paul II, Address to doctors of the Italian Pro-Life Movement, 12 October 1985, in *Insegnamenti di Giovanni Paolo II*, vol. 8/2 (Vatican City: Vatican Polyglot Press, 1985), 933-36; John Paul II, Address to participants in the 2nd International Congress of Food

and Disarmament International, 13 February 1986, in *Insegnamenti*, vol. 9/1:190-92; John Paul II, Address to participants in a Pro-Life Seminar, 1 March 1986, in *Insegnamenti*, vol. 9/1:457-62; John Paul II Address to members of the Italian Pro-Life Movement, 25 January 1986, in *Insegnamenti*, vol. 9/1:562-64; Sacred Congregation for the Doctrine of the Faith, *Declaration on Abortion*, 18 November 1974, *The Pope Speaks* 19 (1974):250-62.

11. The texts of the church's magisterium on artificial insemination are: Pius XII, "Medical Ethics," 29 September 1949, *Catholic Mind* 48 (1950):250-53; Pius XII, "Apostolate of the Midwife"; Pius XII, "Marriage and Parenthood," 19 May 1956, in *The Pope Speaks* 3 (New York: Pantheon Books, 1957), 191-97; Pius XII, "Moral Questions of Heredity," 12 September 1958, in *The Pope Speaks* 6 (New York: Pantheon Books, 1960), 392-400; John Paul II, "The Person Is the Measure of Everything Human"; John Paul II, Address to members of the World Medical Association, 29 October 1983, *Origins* 13 (1983):385-89. The texts of the magisterium on the inseparability of the two aspects of the conjugal act are: Pius XII, "Marriage and Parenthood," 19 May 1956, *Gaudium et Spes*, 50-51; *Humanae Vitae*, 10-12; John Paul II, *Familiaris Consortio*, 32a-32b; John Paul II, "Il Rispetto per l'Opera di Dio nella sua Varietà e Ricchezza," 21 November 1984, and "Nell'atto Coniugale le Finalità Unitiva e Procreativa Sono," 11 July 1984, in D. Tettamanzi, ed., *Matrimonio e Famiglia nel Magistero della Chiesa* (Milan: Massimo, 1986), 498 and 458-80.

12. D. Tettamanzi, *Bambini Fabbricati* (Casale Monferrato: Piemme, 1985); M. Zalba, "Aspetti Morali e Giurídici circa la Inseminazione Artificiale," *Palestra del Clero* (1985); R. Garcia de Haro, "Recondazione Artificiale," *Studi Cattolici* (1984); C. Caffarra, "La Fecondazione in Vitro: Problemi Etici," *Medicina e Morale* 1(1985):67-71.

13. J. Visser, "Problemi Etici dell'Embryo Transfer," *Università degli Studi di Milano* 8-9 (1982-1983):1-171; G.B. Guzzetti, "Fecondazione In Vitro e Morale," *Federazione Medica* 27 (1984):13-19; G. Perico, *Problemi di Etica Sanitaria* (Milan: Ancora, 1986), 215-36.

14. *Gaudium et Spes*, 15.

15. *Dei Verbum*, in W.M. Abbott, ed., *Documents of Vatican II* (New York: Guild Press, 1966), 10.

16. *Humanae Vitae*, 4; D. Tettamanzi, *Bambini Fabricati*, 147-56; S. Pinckaers and C. Josaphat Pinto de Oliviera, eds., *Universalité et permanence des Lois Morales* (Fribourg: Presses Universitaires, 1986).

17. John Paul II, Address to participants in the National Conference of the Pontifical Commission for the Apostolate of Health Care Workers, 24 October 1986, *Medicina e Morale* 1-3 (1987):168-71.

18. Ibid.

19. Other magisterial documents referred to in the Instruction are *Gaudium et Spes*, 24 and 51: "Therefore when there is question of harmonizing conjugal love with the responsible transmission of life, the moral aspect of any procedure does not depend solely on sincere intentions or on evaluation of motives. It must be determined by objective standards. These, based on the nature of the human person and his acts, preserve the full sense of mutual self-giving and human procreation in the context of true love." Various authors have underlined this connection, creation-procreation in reference to spousal love: Tettamanzi, *Bambini Fabricati*, 61-77; C. Ghidelli, "L'Insegnamento Biblico sul Dono della Vita," 51-71; T.P. Doyle, *The Moral Inseparability of Unitive and Procreative Aspects of Human Sexual Intercourse* (St. Louis: Pope John Center, 1984), 261-86.

20. See also P. Ramsey, *Fabricated Man: The Ethics of Genetic Control* (New York: Haven, 1970); G. Perico, "Fecondazione Umana Extracorporea," *Aggiornamenti Sociali* 20 (1969):235ff; G. Perico, "Fecondazione Extracorporea ed Embryo Transfer," *Aggiornamenti Sociali* 35 (1984):257-70; J. Schmitt, "Biologie: Jusqu'où Peut on Aller?" *Le Point* (1984):46; W.E. May, "Begotten, Not Made: Further Reflections on the Laboratory Generation of Human Life," *International Review of Natural Family Planning* 10(1986):1-22.

21. B.M. Ashley, *Theologies of the Body: Humanist and Christian* (Braintree, Mass.: The Pope John Center, 1985); L.F. Badia and R.A. Sarno, *Morality: How to Live It Today* (New York: Alba House, 1980); G. Gatti, "Il Significato del Corpo in Etica Sessuale," in *Attualità della Teologia Morale* (Rome: Università Urbaniana, 1987), 267-83; J. Gevaert, *Problema dell'Uomo* (Leumann, Elle DiCi, 1984); R.M. Hogan, *Covenant of Love: John Paul II on Sexuality, Marriage and Family in the Modern World* (Garden City, N.Y.: Doubleday, 1985); F. Giunchedi, *Etica e Scienze Umane* (Naples: Dehoniane, 1985); T. Goffi and G. Piana, eds., *Corso di Morale*, vol. 2, *Diakonia* (Brescia: Queriniana, 1983); A. Gunthor, *Chiamata e Risposta*, vol. 3 (Rome: Paoline, 1984); B. Häring, *Liberi e Fedeli in Christo*, vol. 2 (Rome: Paoline, 1980); L. Lorenzetti, *Trattato di Etica Teologica*, vol. 2 (Bologne: Dehoniane, 1981); B. Melchiorre, *Il Corpo* (Brescia: La Scuola, 1984); G. Rossi, "Il Rapporto Uomo-Donna," in Lorenzetti, ed., *Trattato di Etica Teologica*, 399-458; J. Sarano, *Essai sur la Signification du Corps* (Paris: Paoline, 1975); M.F. Schwartz et al., eds., *Sex and Gender: A Theological and Scientific Inquiry* (St. Louis: The Pope John Center, 1984); S. Spinsanti, *Corpo nella Cultura Contemporanea* (Brescia: Queriniana, 1983); D. Tettamanzi, "La Sessualità Umana: Prospettive Antropologiche, Etiche e Pedagogiche," *Medicina e Morale* 2 (1984):129-54; M. Vidal, *L'Atteggiamento Morale: Etica della Persona* (Assisi: Cittadella, 1979); X. Zubiri, *Problema dell'Uomo* (Palermo: Augustinus, 1985); D. Tettamanzi, "Fecondazione Artificiale e Immagine della Famiglia," in Sgreccia, ed., *Il Dono della Vita*, 123-45; D. Tettamanzi, "Il Procreare Umano e la Fecondazione in vitro," *Medicina e Morale* 2 (1986):347-67; K. O'Rourke, O.P., "Scienze e Technologie Nuove," *Dolentium Hominum* 5 (1987):44-55; B. Honings, "Il Fattibile non e' Sempre Agibile," *Dolentium Hominum* 5 (1987):55-59; C. Caffarra, "La Transmissione della Vita Umana nella 'Familiaris Consortio'," *Medicina e Morale* 2 (1983); C. Martelet, *Amore Coniugale e Rinnovamento Conciliare* (Assisi: Cittadella, 1968); R. Garcia de Haro, "La Fecondazione Artificiale," *Studi Cattòlici* (1984):272ff; A. Rodriguez Luno and R. Lopez Mondejar, *La Fecondazione In Vitro: Aspetti Etici e Morali* (Rome: Città Nuova Editrice, 1986); K. Wojtyla, *Amore e Responsabilità* (Torino: Merutti, 1969); *Persona e Atto* (Vatican: Libreria Editrice Vaticana, 1982); K. Wojtyla, "La Visione Antropològica della 'Humanae Vitae'," *Lateranum* 44 (1978):125-45; F. Giunchedi, "La Fecondazione In Vitro: Considerazioni Morali," *Rassegna di Teologia* 24 (1983):289-307; F. Giunchedi, "Considerazione: Morali Sulla Fecondazione Artificiale," *Civiltà Cattòlica* 1(1984):223-41; The Bishops' Joint Committee on Bioethical Issues, *Medicina e Morale* 4 (1983):435-48; B. Honings, "La Fivet," in *Attualità della Teologia Morale* (Rome: Università Urbaniana, 1987), 249-83.

LISA SOWLE CAHILL, Ph.D.

What Is the "Nature" of the Unity of Sex, Love and Procreation? A Response to Elio Sgreccia

It is clear to me that the agreements between Msgr. Sgreccia and myself are both numerous and more fundamental than our disagreements. The same can be said of the conclusions of the recent Vatican Instruction, which I and most other Roman Catholics would follow in affirming both a duty to treat the embryo with respect, and the rightful place of parenthood within marriage. Msgr. Sgreccia also offers a cogent critique of Western cultural attitudes toward technology, discerning an overemphasis on human freedom and control, and an overreliance on technology to resolve human problems. Certainly agreement on these points, which are quite "countercultural" in the Western twentieth century context, offers a base of Catholic unity in the analysis of reproductive technologies which is much more important than practical differences about how the value of the embryo and the unity of parenthood and spousehood might best be realized concretely.

Msgr. Sgreccia also rightly encourages us to press our practical analysis of infertility therapy back to the foundational levels, and to build toward a positive dialogue about its practical applications.

As a contribution to such a dialogue, I would like to add three questions for consideration. I will outline these very briefly, then develop them in turn. (1) Are there some *positive values* or insights contributed by modern culture in relation to the human person, and if so, what are they? How do they bear on church teaching about reproductive technologies? (2) Among the basic

theological-ethical considerations, what is the contemporary
meaning of the *"natural law"* methodology itself? A natural law
approach to moral analysis continues to be a distinctive contribution of Roman Catholic ethics. (3) When we enter into the
dialogue for which Msgr. Sgreccia calls, how is that process
undertaken? How does it reflect on our understanding of what
the natural law is, and of how the natural law is known?

I. Culture and Its Contributions

I am impressed by the predominantly negative language of
the first part of Msgr. Sgreccia's paper. The modern attitude
toward human life and technology is described in terms of
"domination and manipulation," and even "destruction." It is
"Promethean." It is summed up by the declaration attributed to
Oppenheimer, "We are working for the devil."[1] Given this
interpretation of the audience to which the Instruction is directed,
the meaning of the Instruction itself becomes an exercise in
negativity—a negation of the negations.

But are there positive contributions of the modern view of the
person, of history, and of morality? Can the teaching of the
church learn from these contributions and build on them? I
would suggest that at least three contributions are relevant. (1)
Contemporary thought offers a self-consciously historical understanding of the person, of cultures, and of knowing. A "historical"
understanding must be distinguished carefully from a "historicist"
understanding. Moral evaluation aims for transcendence of the
particular situation, decision and act—hence it is possible to speak
of "objectivity" in ethics. Nonetheless, all moral evaluation (even
within church teaching) is historically rooted. Historicity must not
be seen merely as a negative limit to the potential universality
of substantive moral claims, but as the very condition of possibility
of community, hence language, hence philosophy. The historical
contextualization of experience and reflection on experience give
them their intelligibility. It is from the concreteness of experience
that we derive moral insights and are able to generalize moral
claims. It is through dialogue among moral, religious, and cultural
communities that we test and improve our moral formulations and

make them more inclusive (i.e., more "universal"). (2) Historical self-consciousness leads us to an appreciation of concrete experience as a testing ground and also a point of renewal for philosophical interpretation of spheres of experience such as sexuality, marriage, and parenthood. (3) A final insight is suggested by Msgr. Sgreccia himself, in his comment that contemporary culture is sensitive to the value of liberty.[2] Although often individualist, our culture is at least appreciative of freedom as a crucial element in human dignity and morality, an appreciation which is at the very basis of the Instruction's own call for equal respect for all persons. Of course, part of our ethical task is to determine more precisely when the proper exercise of human freedom crosses the border into excess, or indeed into the "domination" which Msgr. Sgreccia deplores. However, the basic recognition of human freedom, as an integral part of human dignity, is reflected in modern personalist philosophy, so influential in the writings of John Paul II, particularly on marriage and sexual expression. The call of *Humanae Vitae* for "responsible parenthood"[3] testifies that control over reproduction is not bad in itself. The issues, rather, are ones of means and limits. Of course, this question cannot be settled precisely nor with nuance if we simply object to all control, or use terms such as "domination" and "manufacture" without drawing careful lines. The question before us is that of the proper understanding and role of human freedom in sexuality, marriage, and parenthood. If the "law" of the "nature" of the human person in these matters is known by reasonable reflection on experience, then the formulations of the magisterium have constantly to be brought back to concrete reality, to the experience of couples and parents, and to the nuances of cultural contexts which may pose old questions in new ways.

A key ingredient in the contemporary Western moral understanding of sex and marriage is an enhanced appreciation of the fact that it is the interpersonal relationship of the couple which is at the heart of marriage. This emphasis on relationship is closely aligned with the modern Western valuation of individual dignity and freedom. Current magisterial teaching on sex and marriage has appropriated this focus on the affective relationship of the couple. In the more traditional views which have shaped basic church teaching on the subject (for instance, through the writings of Thomas Aquinas), the social and economic functions of marriage and family were much more prominent. Hence the primacy of procreation, not only in "justifying" sexual acts themselves, but even more in enhancing the size, continuity, economic productivity, and social influence of the family. The personal relationship of the spouses might develop over time (into a "friendship," as Thomas put it), but it was unlikely to be the major incentive for entering the married state. However, in the recent Catholic tradition—in Vatican II's *Gaudium et Spes*, Paul VI's *Humanae Vitae*, and John Paul II's "personalist" writings and lectures on marriage and sexuality—the relation of the spouses moves to center stage. A familiar example of this general shift is the language of the 1983 Code of Canon Law, in which that to which spouses give consent is the *consortium*, the partnership of the whole of life. This language contrasts sharply with the 1917 Code's understanding of consent as directed toward the "right over one another's body" for the acts ordained to procreation.[4] It represents increased recognition of the personal spousal relationship.

Stated succinctly, the general contemporary Catholic view is that *marriage is a partnership which should be characterized above all by mutual love, which is expressed sexually, and which is conducive to children.* In magisterial statements, this fundamental definition is expressed and protected by a basic (and "absolute") sexual norm which defines procreation and the love or unity of the couple as the natural and morally obligatory purposes of sexual acts. As articulated in *Humanae Vitae*, and in the Instruction, the inseparable unity of these ends is to be maintained in each and every sexual act. Further, this unity is thought to entail certain specific prohibitions: against artificial birth control, conception without sexual acts, sexual acts outside marriage, and reproduction outside marriage.

We may note that such moral norms tend to focus our understanding of sexual morality once more on sexual acts, rather than on the relation of the couple. Can it be said that the inherent nature of the marriage relationship demands all these particular norms? Or is a pronounced focus on proper and improper acts more at home in (and a product of) the traditional view of marriage and procreation? In the latter view, the natural physiological reproductive outcome was also morally most significant, and close supervision of sexual activity was necessary to safeguard social and family interests in births. Some social and moral concern about the proper structure and sphere of sexual acts is understandable, since it is clear that uncontrolled and uninstitutionalized sexual acts are in any society a source of significant social and moral problems. Hence there is a certain legitimacy to the standard Christian stress on *control* of sexuality and reproduction. Even so, social control of sexuality does not amount to an adequate morality of either marriage or parenthood if the interpersonal dimensions of sexuality are appreciated positively.

If the relationship of the married couple were to be given sustained and serious attention in its own right, and independently of any stake in defending or disputing current magisterial teaching, what moral norms would the marital experience yield (assuming that "an" experience could be inferred from the many cultural variations on the theme)? If we were to test sexual and parental norms in the experiences of marriage and family, which of the traditional ones would be affirmed? How are sex and procreation related experientially to the love of the couple? What role do and should sexual acts play in the spousal and parental *relationships*? Can we distinguish an ideal relation of love, sex and procreation from imperfect but morally acceptable compromises, arising from less than ideal situations? What would a morally acceptable compromise on these issues look like? Are there any values which no acceptable compromise can afford to set aside?

I suggest that the movement from procreative acts to personal relationship in the Roman Catholic teaching about the nature of marriage represents a "paradigm shift" which is still incompletely reflected in Catholic sexual ethics. The first feature of the emerging paradigm is that the partnership of the couple is the basic category; the partnership opens out onto family and society. (The moral question to be addressed here is that of the role of sex and procreation in expressing and maintaining this relationship and its broader contribution.) The second feature of the new paradigm is that the biological structure of a sexual act is secondary to (not absent from) its moral meaning. (The major virtue of "Natural Family Planning" is that it emphasizes the total relationship of the couple, and does not hang its whole weight from a negative attack on artificial interference with the structure of sexual acts.)

Once the shift is recognized, then acts must be evaluated in the context of the marital relationship. For instance, acts of procreation which rely on a procreative partner outside the marriage are morally questionable because they seem to make the desire to procreate more important than the fundamental marital partnership, and bring a third party (via shared parenthood) into the nexus of basic human relationships which marriage is supposed to support and protect. However, artificial assistance to conception within marriage, even when it circumvents sexual union, only makes sexual union secondary to the shared goal of parenthood and to the partnership of the spouses. I do not believe that, experientially, most married persons would rank particular sexual acts with their spouses on a par with their total love relationship or their shared relation to their children.

Physical goods and values can have an important relation to human relationships, but they are expressive and contributory, rather than fundamentally constitutive of such relationships. Msgr. Sgreccia argues, for instance, that in IVF, "Procreation is not closely related to the *act* of conjugal love but to the biologist's *technical activity*."[5] I would say, rather, that both the act of love and the technology of conception should be related to the marital partnership of the couple. An act of conception should not be considered as an entity apart, with a moral character which can be understood independently of this relationship. If there is an inviolable value in the triad of love, sex, and procreation, it is clearly the value which is in and of itself a personal one: love. Indeed, how could it be claimed that the other two values are on a par with this one, and not expressions which proceed from it? An each-and-every-act analysis of the "inseparability" of sex, love and procreation distorts the valid unity among them by tying that unity to specific sexual acts rather than to the marital relationship. The corporeal aspects of marriage and parenthood must be subsumed under the interpersonal meanings in order to have moral intelligibility.

The problem before us—not here resolved—is to give an experientially true definition of the relation between the physical and the affective, cognitive, and volitional aspects of spousehood and parenthood. Then we must define more carefully the limits on freedom which are required by biological relationships. To say that biology sets all the limits or can never set limits at all is, I think, to adopt a dualist anthropology, in which the person as spirit or freedom is severed from the personal as corporeity or body.

Biology sets a rightful limit only when a biological act or intervention entails an inappropriate involvement of the person whose "biology" is in question. Thus biological manipulation of one (or both) of two persons already within a morally good relationship (marriage), in order to further a proper end of that relationship (procreation), is morally acceptable. It does not distort or change the basic personal relationship within which procreation is accomplished biologically: marriage. This remains true even if that accomplishment entails a biomedical replacement for sexual intercourse in the process of conception. The manipulation of reproductive biology still remains within the parameters of an appropriate and morally valid reproductive relationship of persons. Moral inappropriateness is indicated at least in cases in which the ostensible justification of some "purely biological" act is contingent on our ability to deny any significant connection at all of the person as a whole with that aspect of his or her biology which is to be involved. If dualism is a requisite maneuver in the justification of a "biological" act, then both the justifying process and the act are suspect.

I would set a limit in procreative technologies at the use of gametes of persons from outside the marriage in order to accomplish the procreative project of the couple. These methods are premised on a preconceived intention of the donor to sever the activity of procreation from the personal relation of parenthood (vis-à-vis both the offspring and the procreative partner). The recipients endorse and support this separation, perhaps even offering payment. From a nondualist perspective, I think it must be concluded, first, that third-party methods of obtaining ova or sperm intrude a third *person* on the marriage, even if he or she is supposedly affectively uninvolved and is recognized only as a biological contributor. Second, to create deliberately a reproductive situation in which any *prima facie* connection between genetic and social parenthood is from the outset denied and suppressed is again to treat dualistically a fundamental and powerful relationship of the human *person*. In third party methods, the parties act as though there were no morally important relation of genetic reproduction either to a marital or a parental personal relation.

II. Natural Law

Msgr. Sgreccia quotes the Instruction as teaching, "Science and technology require, for their own intrinsic meaning, an unconditional respect for the fundamental criteria of the moral law: that is to say, they must be at the service of the human person, of his inalienable rights, and his true and integral good according to the design and will of God."[6] This statement raises two key questions: (1) How is the moral law known? (2) How is it related to faith? Or, how is it related to the role of the magisterium as religious interpreter of natural law, a role addressed at length by Msgr. Sgreccia?[7]

Basic assets of the natural law method of moral argument are that it establishes an *objective moral order*, confidence in the ability of human *reason* to know that order, and the existence of a *community of moral discourse* in which persons and groups from different religious and cultural traditions can join in the discovery of moral values and norms. I would suggest that if the interpretation of natural law that the church proposes relies too heavily on authority and not enough on the careful construction of a reasonable consensus about basic human values, then the church's effectiveness as moral teacher (especially in policy matters) will be undercut severely.

Thomas Aquinas, Catholicism's model for natural law philosophy, tells us that, although the principles of the speculative reason "contain the truth without fail," "The practical reason, on the other hand, is busied with contingent matters, about which human actions are concerned: and consequently, although there is necessity in the general principles, the more we descend to matters of detail, the more frequently we encounter defects." And, "in matters of action, truth or practical rectitude is not the same for all, as to matters of detail, but only as to the general principles: and where there is the same rectitude in matters of detail, it is not equally known to all."[8] New reproductive technologies are preeminently "contingent matters." The applicable principle is undisputed: unity of love, sex, and procreation. But the applications in this area have to be seriously considered, and with care and nuance. We need courage to criticize, or as Msgr. Sgreccia says, "prophesy." But also needed are caution and humility in formulating specific moral guidelines. The church needs to look more broadly and more sympathetically at the diverse experiences of those engaged in the "contingent matters" in question. These include married couples, especially parents and infertile couples; and those medical professionals involved in specialties such as marriage and family counseling, embryology, obstetrics and infertility therapy.

III. The Process of Dialogue

Msgr. Sgreccia calls for a process of exploration of these issues. He tells us that the moralist has a "double task": to "investigate more deeply the reasons given by the magisterium to support the ethical indications," and to make the teaching *"accessible* to our contemporaries through a positive effort of mediation."[9] I would go further than this, in two ways. First, it is not as if moral theology, or even the magisterium, is in possession of a timeless and quite specific set of moral rules regarding artificial reproduction, which it must now translate in the language "accessible" to our "contemporaries." Moral understanding of values to be protected and rules specifying them can arise only out of an interaction among several sources: contemporary experience, including empirical science and medicine; the tradition of the church, including Scripture, theology, and magisterium; and refined philosophical analysis, in which religious persons and teachers may cooperate with others in arriving at a better understanding of what the natural law demands in any particular area of moral practice. Second, historical and cultural contextualization is absolutely crucial in order to communicate any moral message at all. Joseph Fuchs has spoken to this point:

Revelation itself, and even more so tradition and the magisterium, already adhere to some theological assertions which
are formulated as propositions. We should not forget, however,
that these assertions are always necessarily formulated in the
language of a particular horizon of thought, with its own way
of posing questions. We have need not only of interpretation
but also of a hermeneutic, in order correctly to translate into
contemporary ways of questioning and understanding those
things put differently in the sources of our faith and in the
theology (theologies) of times past. Only in this way can we
guarantee a genuine transmission of the content of our faith,
and not just a verbal correctness which could produce a
falsification or an inexact rendering of the tradition.[10]

To mention a specific example of the process of reconsidera-
tion of moral teachings in view of the needs of particular historical contexts, John T. Noonan has argued that the tradition's
prohibition of artificial contraception was founded on a need to
protect the five values of marital love, dignity of the spouses,
goodness of sexuality, value of procreation, and education of
children. But the prohibition may not be as effective a means of
protecting these very values in our culture as in cultures past.[11]
A new theological, moral, and pastoral perspective on these values
needs to be gained in order to secure them *in their objectivity*, by
means of moral rules which address their relation to concrete
historical dangers and possibilities.

   This, of course, can be accomplished only by means of a
dialogical, sympathetic and nuanced understanding of the setting
in which the values are to be realized. Msgr. Sgreccia repeatedly
characterizes disagreement with the magisterium as "ethical utilitarianism," "relativism," "proportionalism," and so on.[12] We need
nuance at the level of theory as well as of conclusions in morality.
Terms such as the above do not all mean the same thing, nor is
it accurate to paint with such a broad brush all questions which
are posed about traditional moral formulations. As we look for
an appropriate model of communication and dialogue, we might
use profitably the development of Roman Catholic teaching on
social issues. We recognize with increasing clarity that sex, family,
and reproduction are not "personal" issues in any narrow sense,

but raise pressing social questions. Many authors have pointed out that we could hope for greater consistency in the methods of development and the authoritative presentation of church teaching on "personal" questions such as parenthood and "social" questions such as international conflict. I have space only to note that dialogue of the magisterium with Catholics in the North American context would enhance its appreciation of the loud call of Catholic women for full and equal participation with men in the interrelated spheres of family, society, and church. This is an important change in the fundamental context in which questions of marriage and parenthood are formulated.

IV. Conclusions

My basic disagreement with Msgr. Sgreccia regards the moral viability of homologous reproductive technologies. The question properly before us is not whether all medical control of reproduction is immoral, but what are the proper limits and uses of technology in accomplishing reproduction. I see no convincing argument that homologous techniques may not be evaluated as appropriate interventions in the presence of physical abnormalities, to accomplish the unity of love and procreation in the sexually expressed relation of a couple.

I also have several agreements, both explicit and inferred. (1) The procreative relationship of parent to child is undeniably a great and precious good. But it is not an absolute value, one which should be sought at any cost and through any means. (2) Following from this, the love commitment of spouses sets reasonable, humane and Christian parameters in which to undertake parenthood. The partnership of spouses is the humanly appropriate context for childbearing. Thus donor methods are morally problematic. (3) Even within marriage, the use of technology must be judged in relation to the love and commitment of spouses, and by its effects on their relationship. Is the stress of IVF, for example, proportionate to its relatively low success rate? Does IVF technology lift up procreation as a goal to the same extent as did the old ethic in which procreation was the sole motive fully justifying sex? Is there a distortion in both cases? (One also thinks of the many children available internationally for U.S. adoption. The biogenetic relation to one's children is understandably prized—but just how commanding should it be?) (4) The expenditure of social and health care resources on a "high tech" remedy for a few may not meet the test of distributive justice. (5) Experimentation on the embryo, and its production for medical uses, are very real and major problems. They should unite in protection of the embryo both those who do and those who do not see it as a "person" in the full sense from the time of fertilization, and those who do or do not approve IVF in some form. On this as on other issues, secondary points of difference should not obscure major points of unity, nor distract energy from a unified Roman Catholic witness to the intimate relation of sexual expression, parenthood, and the commitment of spouses.

Notes

1. Elio Sgreccia, "Moral Theology and Artificial Procreation in Light of *Donum Vitae*," trans. Cristina Demagistris, this volume, 120.

2. Ibid., 132.

3. Paul VI, *Humanae Vitae* (New York: Paulist Press, 1968), sec. 10.

4. See Canons 1055.1 and 1057.2 of the 1983 Code. For a commentary and comparison with the 1917 Code, see Ladislas Orsy, S.J., *Marriage in Canon Law* (Wilmington, Del.: Michael Glazier, 1986), 54-63.

5. Sgreccia, 122.

6. Sgreccia, 125.

7. Ibid., 127, 128.

8. Thomas Aquinas, *Summa Theologiae*, I-II Q 94 a 1.

9. Sgreccia, 127.

10. Joseph Fuchs, S.J., *Personal Responsibility and Christian Morality* (Washington, D.C.: Georgetown University Press, 1983), 6.

11. John T. Noonan, *Contraception: A History of Its Treatment by the Catholic Theologians and Canonists*, enlarged ed. (Cambridge, Mass.: Harvard University Press, 1986), 533.

12. See, for instance, Sgreccia, 123.

IV.

IMPACT ON LEGISLATION AND PUBLIC POLICY

EDMUND D. PELLEGRINO, M.D.

Donum Vitae, *Part III:*
Three Dilemmas for Americans

I. Introduction

In the first two of its three parts, the Vatican Instruction, also known as *Donum Vitae*,[1] prescribes the moral norms governing the procreation of human life and the modern reproductive technologies associated with it. The Instruction spells out the moral dangers of some of the newer technologies. It encourages continued scientific research provided it always remains responsive to the moral norms of the Catholic Tradition.

In the third of its three parts, the Instruction moves from the guidance of consciences to legislative intervention. It rejects reliance on the conscience of scientific investigators to safeguard the dignity of the embryo, of marriage and the family, and the unity of the procreative act. It calls for legislation that will regulate reproductive technologies in conformity with the teachings of the Catholic Church. And, if such interventions fail, the Instruction advises conscientious objection and passive resistance to laws and policies that threaten human life "in its origins" as well as the "dignity of procreation."

The third part of the Instruction raises several serious unresolved dilemmas for Catholics and their fellow citizens living in morally heterogeneous, democratic societies like the United States. Three of these dilemmas seem of particular interest to Americans at this time.

First, is the dilemma of religious liberty and its limits. To what extent may any religious group inject its beliefs into the formulation of civil laws, without violating the religious freedom of those who do not share those beliefs? Is the right to religious liberty for Catholics predicated on the assumption that believers refrain from imposing their beliefs on others by law? Does this mean that religious beliefs are de facto excluded from legislative action? Are such beliefs simply private matters without implication for the larger society?

Second, is the dilemma of conscience and consensus in ethics. In democratic, morally pluralist societies, some form of public consensus is required to formulate legislation. Does this necessitate consensus as the only means for resolving conflicts of moral values? What is the relationship between consensus based in natural law, which is consistent with Catholic teaching, and consensus based on majority vote?

Third, is the dilemma of Catholic belief and political action in secular societies. Catholics have an obligation in conscience to take the teachings of the church authority seriously. At the same time they have obligations to live peaceably and to participate fully and effectively as citizens of the large society which may reject some of the most fundamental Roman Catholic beliefs about human life—precisely those beliefs which are the concern of the Instruction.

These three dilemmas are particularly pertinent for Catholics living in the United States. Here, current public opinion is increasingly secular or libertarian in tone, biomedical ethics has become largely procedural rather than substantive, and public opinion runs strongly against the legislation of morality. If Roman Catholics are to implement their beliefs about human life, beliefs which they hold binding on all humans, they face conceptual and practical questions whose answers are not yet fully formulated.

II. The Dilemma of Religious Liberty

The Instruction arrives on the American scene at a sensitive time in the history of the relationship between religious belief and public life. On the one hand, many Americans believe our country is still a "Christian" nation and that Christian values must shape public policy and law if the national moral lassitude they perceive is to be cured. On the extreme other hand, many see any intrusion of religious values into civic life as an assault on individual freedoms and therefore as politically retrogressive and lethal to any genuine conception of freedom in a secular society. In between, there are growing numbers of believers and nonbelievers who respect the values of religion but who are convinced that people should be free to make their own decisions about abortion, euthanasia, in vitro fertilization, etc.

These divisions were evident in the last two presidential campaigns of 1984 and 1988. In the political debates, we heard from fundamentalists who would mold American life along scriptural lines, centrists who hold to their own personal religious beliefs but would refrain from imposing them on others by law, and militant secularists who would exclude religion entirely and deprive churches and their institutions of tax exempt status.[2]

In these debates, Catholics themselves were divided on the extent to which their beliefs, even on so vital an issue as abortion, should be the subject of legislative action or determinative of their choice of candidates. Some American bishops chastised Catholic candidates who chose to separate their personal beliefs from their political stance.[3] Other Catholics placed the abortion issue above every other consideration and made abortion the test of political support. Some believed that attempts to reverse *Roe v. Wade* should be limited to legal means. Others felt impelled to active disruption of abortion clinics. Clearly, while Americans are agreed on the importance of religious liberty, they are sharply divided on the degree to which that liberty can be used to shape civic law and public policy.

The dilemma must be confronted in the face of the greatest moral heterogeneity in the history of our country. Our nation has always been morally pluralistic. But until the last few decades the spectrum of moral diversity was limited. At the beginning of the twentieth century, Judeo-Christian values were still thought to be the foundations for American life, both private and public. We might differ in our application of those values but there was little argument that a common set of values did exist. Now, as the twentieth century closes, the range of moral diversity has expanded greatly. It now extends from Fundamentalist Christianity, Orthodox Judaism and Roman Catholicism, to the beliefs of Islam, the religions and philosophies of the Far East and to the extremes of secularism—atheism and even satanism. Indeed, if we examine demographic trends for the twenty-first century, it is possible that adherents to Judeo-Christian values may well become a minority in the United States.[4]

As the spectrum of diversity has widened, the possibilities of any true moral consensus have diminished proportionally. Shared religious values and goals have been superseded by the values and goals of secular democracy. Freedom of choice, freedom to practice one's own values, and mutual respect have become the primary foci of ethical discourse. As a result, the tenor of American moral life is toward moral privatization, relativism, and moral neutrality, both in public and private life. Many of the "human values" that have traditionally been associated with Christian humanism, e.g. compassion, good works, etc., have been expropriated by secular humanists. Judeo-Christian ethical principles have been detached from their theological roots and given the benediction of secular humanism or liberal political philosophy. Ethics without theology is the creed of secular humanists.

The Instruction confronts this milieu of controversy, confusion, and doubt with an uncompromising stand on the most sensitive issues of all, the procreation of human life, the sanctity of the human family in which life is nurtured, and respect for human life in all its forms. The message of the Instruction is clear and unequivocal. It is based in a firm view of human nature, its meaning and destiny. It promulgates a set of moral norms derived from natural law, as well as theological and ecclesiastical teachings.

A substantive body of public opinion and public policy in the United States is manifestly in conflict with the moral norms promulgated by *Donum Vitae*. Since *Roe v. Wade*,[5] Roman Catholic and prochoice advocates have been involved in heated confrontations both in court and in front of abortion clinics. Each year, prolife Catholics stage a "march for life" in Washington, D.C. In April 1989, a prochoice rally drew one of the largest crowds of supporters ever to march on the nation's capital. The Supreme Court's decision in *Webster v. Reproductive Health Services* has exacerbated the debate and has cast serious doubt on the future of *Roe v. Wade*.[6,7]

There is also a growing sentiment favoring active voluntary euthanasia in the United States. Although the attempt to put a euthanasia referendum on the 1988 California ballot was unsuccessful, opinion polls show a growing percentage of support among physicians and the general public.[8] This attempt was legally affirmed in the *Bouvia* case in California, to which reference is made in the next section of this essay.

Additional developments promise further to widen the gap between Roman Catholic moral teaching and a growing segment of American public opinion. For example, recently a special advisory committee to the director of the National Institute of Health voted to approve the use of fetal tissue transplants from electively aborted fetuses.[9] The four dissenting committee members were representatives of two religious traditions: three were Roman Catholics and one a Jewish rabbi. Approval is also now being given by various bodies for research on the "pre-embryo."[10] Withdrawal of artificial nutrition and hydration is sanctioned by the American Medical Association[11] while it is condemned by a committee of the Pontifical Academy of Sciences and the New Jersey Conference of Bishops.[12] In vitro fertilization, specifically condemned by the Instruction, is commonplace. Even the possibility of involuntary active euthanasia of severely handicapped infants and children has been suggested.[13]

Within this climate, the Instruction is seen by many non-Catholics and secularists, as well as some Catholics, as an unwarranted intrusion of church dogma into the life of a democratic society which is built on a "wall" of separation between the religious and secular spheres. Others who may agree with the moral norms promulgated by the Instruction nonetheless feel that the imposition of its recommendations by legislation would undermine free choice. Their views parallel the thinking of some Roman Catholics who consider abortion morally illicit but believe that the question is ultimately a matter of individual conscience.[14]

Religious liberty was woven into American political philosophy from the first establishment of our Republic.[15] It is associated with tolerance for the widest spectrum of personal beliefs and practices. In the documents of Vatican II, religious liberty is strongly and cogently defended as well.[16] Catholics appreciate that religious liberty is essential to the sustenance and growth of the church's salvific and evangelical missions. It is the right of religious liberty that permits the American church to emerge as a significant force in American life. The sympathetic responses to the statements of the American bishops on nuclear war and the economy so clearly depend upon the freedom to teach and publicize religious doctrine.[17]

Is this religious liberty contingent on keeping religious beliefs out of the formulation and legislation of public law and policy? Should religious believers in public office be disenfranchised when they participate in policy formulation on such charged issues as abortion, euthanasia, embryo experimentation, or fetal tissue transplantation? Are arguments based in religious norms of morality simply "political" or "stifling" of medical progress?[18] What if it is held, as the Catholic church holds, that the moral norms it espouses on these issues are grounded in natural law and therefore binding on all persons, Catholic or not? How far beyond persuasion can Catholics go in promulgating their beliefs?

Given the troublous moral climate in American life, the third part of the Instruction could widen the gap between Roman Catholics and many of their fellow Americans. If Catholics implement the dictates of the Instruction in the public arena, do they risk violating the sincerely held beliefs of those who do not share their moral convictions? American Catholics in positions of professional and public authority face a particularly distressing choice. By virtue of their offices they must enforce the laws of the land, yet they cannot violate the law of conscience. Must they withdraw from public life? How far can they go in using public office to advance what they believe to be morally right and good?

Answers to these questions may vary from country to country, with the number of Catholics in the population, the degree of their acceptance of ecclesiastical authority, and their positions in professional and public life. Wisely, the Instruction refrains from precise delineation of the means whereby legislative interventions may be effected. Much therefore is left open for debate and discussion among, and between, Roman Catholics and their fellow citizens.

In countries nominally Catholic in which legislators and policy makers are Catholic, legislative interventions may be easier. This may be the context for the Instruction's use of a term such as "public authorities." In the United States, "public authorities" would have to operate under a legislative mandate arrived at through the democratic process. But even in countries with a Catholic majority, the separation between the temporal and spiritual domains is widening. In countries like the United States without an established or clearly dominant religion, the problems are politically more intricate. They center on the notion of religious liberty and the mutuality of respect for other people's beliefs on which religious liberty depends.

The obvious practical political difficulties of implementing Part III of the Instruction do not provide a justifiable excuse for accommodation to the prevailing mores. However difficult, Catholics must try to find the balance between their obligations as citizens of both the city of God and the city of men.

The issues are not confined to the interests of Roman Catholics. Other religious groups, often holding values in conflict with Roman Catholic moral thinking, are also bound in conscience to have a say in the formulation of public policy. Like Roman Catholics, they too must confront the paradoxes of religious liberty in secular, morally pluralistic democratic societies. The problem raised by *Donum Vitae* is generic for believers in any free and democratic society.

What is abundantly clear from the pragmatic political point of view is that abuse of any liberty, even religious liberty, if it threatens the public order, will end by being itself restricted. Before religious liberty was recognized as a basic human right, tyrannical governments imposed the state religion on their citizens and persecuted dissidents. The paradox now is that religious liberty itself is viewed by those who do not hold such beliefs as a potential restriction on the rights of nonbelievers. For nonbelievers, the doctrines of political liberalism and libertarianism have quasi-religious status. For them, religiously inspired legal restrictions would be perceived in the same light as religious persecution.

We shall return to this dilemma in the last section of this essay.

III. The Dilemma of "Consensus Ethics"

When humans differ in their fundamental beliefs they may resolve conflicts either by violence or peaceable dialogue. Democracies are based in the conviction that peaceable discussion, majority decision and protection of the minority are morally justifiable, while the use of violent suppression of contrary opinions is not.

"Consensus" may be arrived at either by majority vote or by appeal to some common ground of values. When consensus is sought in questions of an essentially moral nature—as in the case of the human life issues that are the concern of *Donum Vitae*—we may speak loosely, to be sure, of "consensual ethics."

"Consensual ethics" may take two forms, a secular version which is based in majority rule and a natural law version based in the appeal to some set of values common to human nature. Majority rule ethics is the dominant mode in our secular society, while natural law consensus is the method most consistent with Roman Catholic political philosophy. The former has serious conceptual difficulties, the latter serious practical difficulties. Both should be examined in some detail as we attempt some resolution of the paradoxes that Catholics face in implementing Part III of the Instruction.

A. Consensus ethics, the secular version

Democratic societies seek to resolve conflict through democratic processes. They turn to public debate, opinion polls, panels of experts, political negotiation, and then to legislation. These processes aim at reaching some consensus, or more accurately, a majority opinion large enough to warrant establishment of a public policy.

These processes are based in a need to advance the public good and maintain public order. They assume that the legitimacy of a government implies consent to abide by its laws. In this way, people with divergent views on what constitutes the best way of life can compromise sufficiently to live and work together peaceably and productively and to mutual advantage. This type of consensus is essential to the political integrity of pluralistic societies. When it is applied, as has been the case in recent years in the United States, to the resolution of moral issues in bioethics, certain conceptual difficulties appear which are especially problematic for Roman Catholics, particularly if they follow the advice of *Donum Vitae*.

The central issue is best epitomized in the comment of a member of the panel convened by the director of the National Institutes of Health to advise on the matter of fetal tissue research and transplantation. Commenting on the irreconcilable differences among panel members on the moral status of the use of tissues obtained from elective abortions, he stated, "where there is no agreement we reach decision by 'consensus'."[19] It is not clear whether he was simply stating a fact or prescribing the procedure he believed most appropriate. He did describe accurately the method increasingly in use in biomedical ethics at the bedside, in hospital and public policy, in the courts and in biological research policies.

Before describing the method of consensus ethics as it is used in these different areas, it is important to point out that the term "consensus" is being used loosely and inaccurately. Consensus etymologically means unanimity, complete agreement, accord, or concordance of opinion among the members of a group.[20] In practice, however, it really means majority vote based not on a common agreement that is unanimous but on the resolution of disagreement in favor of an arbitrarily defined majority. Applied to ethics, consensus ethics is thus really majority vote ethics which overrides differences and indeed sharpens them by dividing a group into "pros" and "cons." It leaves the substantive moral differences intact in the interest of taking an action, or enacting a law. In natural law ethics (*vide intra*), consensus has a different connotation.

We can now examine four examples of the way majority-vote ethics has come to dominate the way decisions are being made in biomedical ethics.

(1) At the bedside

Because of the moral pluralism of American society, conflicts arise frequently at the "bedside" between the participants in medical decisions. The patient, family, physician, nurse, and/or the institution may differ on who should decide and on the criteria to be used. The most common conflicts center on withholding and withdrawing life-sustaining measures, the vigor with which treatment should be pursued, and the place of economics and quality of life of patients who cannot decide for themselves. Religious, cultural, economic and moral values play an important role in the decision. Some may see withdrawal and withholding as morally distinct; some may see them as morally neutral and some as morally wrong. Others distinguish between the administration of food and hydration and mechanical respirators.[21] Some regard any shortening of life even in terminal patients as assisted suicide or premeditated homicide.[22]

When such conflicts occur, resolution is sought through conferences among health team members and patients (and/or their families), or by reference to an ethics committee. First, the participants and health care team members try to agree on a plan of management. If this fails, ethics committees may be invoked. They offer the counsel of an interprofessional interdisciplinary group not immediately involved in the decision. Although ethics committees may try sincerely to help the participants make their own decisions, it is difficult not to interpret their recommendations as the "right" thing to do. Families or patients seeking ethical advice are under stress. They are unfamiliar with ethical reasoning, and perhaps uncertain about their own values. They are easily susceptible to the suggestion that "reasonable people" ought to agree. They may make unsuitable moral compromises in order not to offend. For example, a woman's rejection of a therapeutic abortion may be labeled as "irrational." She may even be judged "incompetent" because of her decision. The more distressed and confused the participants to the decision, the more susceptible they are to the danger of subtle coercion to adopt the majority opinion.

There are similar pressures for conformity on the health care team members as well. Once there is "agreement" on a management plan or the ethics committee has given its opinion, many team members feel bound by loyalty to acquiesce. This can create moral conflicts for the health team, or ethics committee members who sincerely disagree with the decision and yet are expected to play a role in its implementation. Withdrawal from the case is usually difficult for nonphysician members of the team. Health professionals who dissent are sometimes subjected to subtle forms of punitive action, e.g. ostracism, loss of promotion, or even loss of employment.

(2) In the policy arena

Conflicts of the same sort may arise in the larger arena of hospital, community, or government policy. Here, the notion of "consensus" is invoked in a way that may place health care professionals in situations of conflict with the dictates of their consciences. For example, a physician might find him or herself in conflict with hospital policies that refuse admission to poor patients or require the physician to transfer a sick patient for economic reasons to another facility. Or the physician might morally object to cost containment policies which entail delaying or withholding needed consultations or tests, or force a patient's untimely discharge because the days allotted by policy or third party payors for a particular disease have been "used up."

Resolutions to this type of conflict are the result of a political "consensus" which consists largely in the convictions of legislators and administrators that economic necessity requires rationing. Physicians are designated as the rationers. As a result, they are placed in positions of ethical conflict: are they primarily agents of the sick person or of the policy? Yet the "consensus" creating the dilemma is more presumptive than actual. The public has no real voice in deciding how much of the gross national product it wishes to devote to health care. Nor is the ethical impact on the physician-patient relationship of making the doctor the "gatekeeper" examined. Despite this, it is widely claimed that we have already reached the point where rationing of health care is necessary.[23]

"Consensus" in the policy arena is a summation of impressions gained through the media, articles, TV talk shows and public and professional conferences. In this way, self-appointed "opinion makers" shape public responses, often with an eye more to the sensational than the factual or the logically defensible. Opinion polls reinforce the "consensus" obtained in this way and the process becomes self-perpetuating. The dangers of this kind of consensus as a basis for ethical decisions hardly need elaboration.

(3) In law

Another arena for consensual decision making in United States society is the court system. Many of the prevalent opinions that make up the presumed consensus about biomedical ethics derive from highly publicized cases. We need mention only a few: *Quinlan,*[24] *Fox,*[25] *Barber,*[26] *Bouvia,*[27] two *Baby Doe* cases,[28,29] and the *Baby M* case.[30] Decisions dealing with the legal and moral "rights" of patients, families and doctors to limit or withdraw life-sustaining measures appear almost weekly. Some of these court decisions are morally sound, others are not.

In the United States, legal decisions are justifiably given great weight. If two or three courts come down with the same decision, a perception of consensus begins to develop. Many people confuse biomedical ethics with law and consider the moral issues resolved by the judge's decisions. Elsewhere, V. A. Sharpe and I have analyzed the moral reasoning in some of these cases, particularly at the appellate level.[31] We point out the precariousness of judicial opinions in resolving ethical disputes.

Court cases do air the issues and generate public debate. However, they may or may not reflect a genuine consensus. Indeed, in court cases we often see a reversal of the old adage "consensus fecit legem." Instead, the court decision often comes first and the consensus follows. This seems to have been the case in *Roe v. Wade,* if one examines chronologically and conceptually the interaction between public opinion and the Supreme Court's decision.[32] This phenomenon is likely to be repeated if voluntary and involuntary active euthanasia become legal.

Another powerful source of unofficial consensus comes from the reports of expert panels. Because many issues are judged too difficult to be grasped by ordinary citizens, we turn, instead, to panels, commissions, task forces, or blue ribbon committees. These mechanisms are necessary and helpful, but again they can result in the perception of general societal agreement when there is only the agreement of the panelists. Most of the time, attention is focused on a summary of panel recommendations. The reasoning and particularly the substance of the debates and dissenting minority opinions are rarely examined.

One current example which is particularly relevant to the issues discussed in *Donum Vitae* shows clearly how consensus has come to mean majority ethics. In its report to the director of NIH, the Human Fetal Tissue Transplantation Research Panel, following the opinion of the majority, concluded that tissues from electively aborted fetuses could be used for therapeutic and research purposes.[33] Those who favored the use of fetal tissue argued that because abortion is legal, the question of abortion was not relevant to the deliberations about tissue use. They argued that the benefits of fetal tissue use are potentially great and that with strict regulation of procurement, isolation of those obtaining consent for the abortion and those who would use the tissues and the prohibition of tissue donation between family members, the use of these tissues would be justified.

Those who opposed, differed on almost every point. Abortion, they argued, is morally unacceptable even if legally permitted. They argued that a mother who has decided to abort a fetus cannot function as its valid surrogate and cannot, therefore, give a valid consent for the use of its tissue. Fetal research cannot be dissociated from abortion, they argued. The beneficial use of fetal tissue could in fact encourage abortions. It would also encourage a symbiotic relationship between abortion and tissue procurement.

The moral arguments among the panelists were irreconcilable. The central moral questions were neither engaged nor disposed of, yet the moral issue was decided by majority vote.

On the other hand, when the underlying moral issues are not as divisive as abortion, the consensus approach can be effective. The President's Commission for the Study of Ethical Problems in Biomedical and Behavioral Research[34] is one example. Over a period of three years from 1980 through March of 1983, the commission issued eleven volumes on some of the most difficult and controversial questions then at issue in biomedical ethics.

Although commission members had differing moral viewpoints, substantial agreement emerged in their reports. Their recommendations, although not universally sanctioned, have received widespread public support and recognition.

Many hope that with the formation of the new Congressional Biomedical Ethics Board and its Biomedical Ethics Advisory Committee, the same process will ultimately resolve current conflicts over the use of fetal tissue in research and transplantation, the withdrawal and withholding of nutrition and hydration, and mapping of the human genome.[35] It is indicative of the degree of controversy and sensitivity of these issues that these bodies have taken so long to be activated. They have barely begun meeting, and already their political and fiscal future is seriously in doubt.

B. Majority opinion ethics: Some philosophical objections

The practice of ethics by majority opinion, attractive as it may be pragmatically, and consistent as it may seem with democratic process, has serious philosophical deficiencies. First, it transforms moral issues into political or statistical problems. It leaves the underlying moral issues unresolved. Religious and philosophical beliefs about moral norms bind in conscience. Individual conscience cannot be replaced by opinion or law.

Second, majority-vote ethics tends to favor procedure over substance. Agreement on what is a morally acceptable process for decision making is more easily obtained than agreement on principles. Agreement on procedure is essential, but proper procedure does not guarantee morally right actions. Ethics by majority vote ends up begging the whole question of which theory of ethics is to be used. It gives utilitarian and consequentialist theories precedence over deontological theories. Consensual ethics based in majority vote encourages relativism, privatism and subjectivism, and ignores the possibility of an objective order of morality. Cultural sociohistoric determinism is given precedence over universalizable, ethical principles.

What is more, consensus ethics reinforces the growing belief that the only function ethics can have in a pluralistic society is conceptual clarification. It assumes there are no moral laws or principles that can bind whole societies. The major function of democracy itself becomes the resolution of conflict. The classical quest for the good community is abandoned. Moral atomism and moral egoism are the inevitable result whenever ethics is thus reduced to a state of normative irrelevance and impotence.

The type of consensual ethics now in practice creates its own morality, as it were. As people engage in debate about an ethical issue they encounter what they perceive to be an already established "consensus." They are then loath to seem odd or perverse by running against the tide. As more people follow the "consensus"—particularly if it is the consensus of "experts," that consensus itself becomes the moral rule. The classical quest of ethics as a guide to becoming a good person is submerged in the effort to be "reasonable," to accommodate, and to go along with the majority. This is particularly true if a "consensus," spurious or not, becomes a law. The moral obligation is to obey a good law and resist a morally bad one, not to obey any law simply because it exists.

Ultimately, consensual ethics may coerce conscience in more direct ways. We see signs of this in the *Bouvia* and *Requena* cases, where courts overrode the ethics of the professions and institutional conscience in promulgating the patient's *absolute* right to decide when to live and when to die.[36,37] If euthanasia, assisted suicide, or involuntary euthanasia becomes law, physicians who oppose such actions may be under enormous pressure from patients. Bureaucratization of law and public policy is inevitable and this will compound the difficulties for those who feel impelled by conscience to disagree.

The assumptions built into ethics by majority vote must be clearly recognized. They do not vitiate efforts to obtain true consensus, i.e. genuine unanimity and agreement on moral procedure or substance. Given the 2500-year-old history of debate over ethical theories, principles, rules, etc., the practical difficulties of arriving at moral consensus cannot be underestimated. The fact cannot be ignored that, in the absence of true consensus on both philosophical and religious ethics, tension between individual conscience and public laws and policies will remain a reality.

Certainly, the alternative of authoritarian imposition of religious beliefs on whole societies is morally reprehensible, even if the policy in question is itself morally defensible. Conscience cannot be replaced by political or religious regimes any more than it can be replaced by majority vote ethics. Individual moral accountability must somehow be balanced with preservation of the public order and the peaceable resolution of divergent moral beliefs. This is the gravest test democracies must face as their populations become morally, ethnically and culturally ever more diverse.

C. Consensus Ethics—The Natural Law Version

There is, in the Roman Catholic tradition, an alternate form of consensus ethics that is not based in majority vote but in natural law theory. Its most eloquent modern spokesman was Fr. John Courtney Murray.[38] His view is adumbrated in Archbishop Quinn's commentary on the implementation of Part III of *Donum Vitae*.[39] In this view, the elements of consensus formation and the rational principles relating civil and moral law are defined in terms of natural law, a law open to reason and binding on all humans as humans.

This form of consensus does not depend upon public opinion, majority vote, expert panels or court decisions. It is a consensus that arises out of the uniqueness of human nature and it summates the dictates of human reason that define human conduct. Natural law binds all humans not by a set of rules for the solution of every moral dilemma but by a set of eternal and immutable truths which command unanimity by their reasonableness, i.e. on the merits of the arguments in their behalf.[40]

Democratic political philosophy owes much to the natural law tradition. The Declaration of Independence speaks of "the Laws of Nature and Nature's God" and of certain "self-evident" truths, thus acknowledging both the natural and the divine laws. The Preamble to our Constitution, while it asserts that law is an expression of the will of the people, nevertheless recognizes a "higher" law which is universal and immutable. Reck identifies this "higher law" to be the natural law.[41] Reck also outlines the transformations during the Enlightenment of natural law as a universal law to a law of natural rights—liberty, property, etc.

Murray has neatly summarized the requirements of a political philosophy based in the natural law: (1) acceptance of the rule of law as reason, and the state as an ethical organism directing us to the virtuous life, not only to the protection of private interests; (2) the community, not the ruler, as the source of political authority; (3) limiting the scope of the ruler to the political realm; (4) agreement of the ruled to be ruled by law; (5) the right of subgroups to autonomous function (principle of subsidiarity); and (6) sharing of the populace in legislation and executive policy.[42]

It was Murray's contention that political and social conflict were unavoidable unless there was consensus on some such set of propositions that would appeal to Catholics, secularists and others. Moreover, while he felt that certain issues were too important to the moral quality of society to be left solely to private choice, he also recognized the necessity to distinguish between private and public morality:

> ...the effort to bring the organized action of politics and the practical art of state craft directly under the control of Christian values that govern personal and familial life is inherently fallacious. It makes a wreckage not only of public policy but of morality itself.[43]

In contrast with majority rule consensus, Father Murray's position on the necessity of a consensus based in natural law is morally and intellectually sound. However, as he foresaw, there are certain trends in contemporary society which make such a consensus increasingly less effective in the resolution of ethical issues with public policy implications.

For one thing, the whole idea of a natural law as a reflection of divine law and as a repository of immutable values is under increasingly heavy attack. Ethicists, philosophers, opinion makers and the public are coming to believe that ethics is historically, culturally or even personally determined. The ideas of evolutionary biology, genetics, and cultural determinism are antipathetic to an objective moral order of any kind. Meanings of the right, the good, and the virtuous are culturally and societally determined. In a word, the entire epistemological and metaphysical underpinning of natural law theory is being dismantled, sometimes even by Roman Catholic thinkers.

On the side of political philosophy, the parallel dismantling has been underway since the Enlightenment. Locke's insistence on natural rights in his second treatise on government[44] has been extrapolated to the limits of moral privatism, individualism and libertarianism. The Aristotelian linkage of ethics, the politics of legislation, and virtue is increasingly denied in political theory and practice. The function of the state, rather than being the pursuit of the just and virtuous life for its citizens, is being reduced to conflict resolution and the preservation of private property and personal freedom.

Finally, the dissociation of natural from divine law, begun by Grotius in the seventeenth century, has eroded the source from which natural law derives its ultimate authority.[45] Natural law can no longer function as the "higher law," to use Reck's phrase, which modulates the sovereign will of the people. Without that modulation, the will of the majority takes on absolute authority. Majority rule, rather than being an instrument for democratic participation, becomes the supreme authority in the resolution of all sorts of conflicts, moral as well as civil.

This is the viewpoint expressed by ethicists like Engelhardt who despair of achieving moral consensus in pluralistic societies.[46] They emphasize freedom of choice, absence of coercion, and community dialogue as the only way to resolve conflicts of moral values so far as public institutions and public policies go. Engelhardt admits that private communities, like churches or Catholic hospitals, can establish a canonical set of agreed-upon values by which to govern their own communities. Catholic hospitals, for example, can forbid abortion, sterilization, euthanasia, or fetal tissue transplantation in their own institutions. But Catholics outside the confines of their own community of belief should not, in Engelhardt's view, intervene by legislation or regulation to limit the free choice of other members of their societies.

We must respect even the wrong conscience—not its conclusions but its operation in other humans of good will who differ with us. We must also behave in accordance with the spirit of the Gospel to act charitably, mercifully and lovingly with those who do not believe as we do and even with those whose actions are in our eyes morally hurtful. We need no new doctrine here but only to recall the difference between sin and the sinner, objectively immoral acts and subjective moral culpability.

This means we must have the courage and the faith necessary to engage in authentic dialogue. Since Vatican II we have improved the quality of that dialogue but we still fail fully to appreciate that we too can learn from dialogue and that humility about our own failures is required. Dialogue does not mean accommodation to secularization, the abandonment of moral distinctions or the acceptance of relativism. To distance ourselves for fear of moral contamination is to abandon our obligation to see that common ground natural law tells us is there. It is also to abandon the opportunity democratic processes offer us to influence legislation so that the dignity of the family, human life and procreation are indeed safeguarded by law.

As a pilgrim people, enmeshed in the vicissitudes of history, as we shall always be, we always live within constraints we may not prefer. We must use the methods a democratic society affords us: freedom of speech, the right to vote, and the right to persuade, to teach and to campaign for our beliefs. We can and must use these processes not merely to resolve conflict but to work for a better society—one which does indeed conform to the natural law rights of individuals and communities.

If we stay within the constraints imposed by the democratic process, secularists cannot rightfully disenfranchise us as voters and as actors on the public policy scene. By patient dialogue we can persuade our fellow citizens that we possess a common human nature, that there is an objective order of morality, that some societies are morally creditable and others not.

To be sure, moral questions are not settled by majority vote or democratic processes. Yet this is the only peaceable way we can arrive at certain kinds of public decisions. It is one thing to resort to a vote in a democratic pluralistic society because this is the only peaceable mechanism we have for resolving a dispute. It is a very

IV. The Dilemma of Catholic Conscience and Political Action

All these trends constitute formidable obstacles to reliance on natural law as the basis for the consensus necessary to effect the legislative intervention advised in *Donum Vitae*. Since Murray's death, society has become more fragmented and morally heterogeneous. Fewer values are shared that might form the basis for a consensus on public policy. If there is anything approaching "consensus" today, it seems to be the agreement that there are few values we can in fact agree upon.

In this atmosphere, Catholics and others who still seek a natural law consensus as the instrument whereby social and moral conflicts are to be resolved are becoming a minority. Natural law ethics, rather than being an appeal to reason and the commonalities of human nature, is interpreted as a rationalization for conforming the whole of public mores to sectarian teachings. Catholics all too often are seen, not as fellow citizens, working for what they believe within the constraints of the democratic process, but as abusers of religious freedom, using that freedom to coerce others into conformity with the teachings of Roman authority.

Formidable and real as these impediments may be, Catholics—as citizens and as Christians—cannot exculpate themselves from the duty to work for a more humane and moral society. In the message of the gospel they have a source of enormous moral power but they must use that power wisely, prudently and with charity. In a pluralistic society under democratic political philosophy, "legislative intervention," as the third part of *Donum Vitae* puts it, can still legitimately be pursued, but only under certain specific conditions.

The first and most difficult condition is to remember those sad times in the church's history when too close an alliance with temporal power led to the violation of human rights of nonbelievers, forced conversions and discrimination. It helps little to point out that the church has always taught that no one is to be converted by coercion. Instead, we must acknowledge and repent for these lapses. If we are to be creditable we would do well to affirm strongly the teaching of Vatican II on the primacy of human conscience in the moral life.[47]

different thing to accept majority vote ethics as determinative of what is right or wrong morally or to abandon all hope of moral consensus. Indeed, the strength of the Catholic tradition is that it has not abandoned the ancient quest of humanity for the right and the good. Others look to us as beacons warning society of the moral shoals toward which a disregard for the dignity of human life will drive us. Witness the approbation given by non-Catholics to the insistence of *Donum Vitae* that biological progress be subjected to moral constraint, even though they might not agree with the ban on in vitro fertilization. Our tradition has always had enormous moral power when we have used it authentically, that is to say, in the spirit of the gospel.

We must work to influence legislation so that laws will not legitimate violations of the dignity of human life and procreation such as abortion, voluntary and involuntary active euthanasia, eugenic manipulation of the human gametocyte, surrogate motherhood or embryo experimentation. These threats to the dignity of human life are also direct threats to the public order and safety. They are inimical to the welfare of the whole society.

On some other matters, those which are more private, in which laws are less enforceable and the threat to the public order and safety is not so clear, it is wiser and ultimately more effective to use persuasion, dialogue, and teaching than to insist on legislation.

Catholics are bound in conscience to take seriously the teachings of *Donum Vitae* and, as citizens, to seek to influence legislation in ways that are effective and convincing to those who do not share Catholic beliefs. All Catholics—physicians, nurses, biological scientists, lawyers, legislators and judges—must know the Catholic position on the human life issues with which *Donum Vitae* deals. They must be prepared to explain its natural law, as well as its theological foundations. They must recognize that the church does not oppose the search for new biological knowledge nor its legitimate use to relieve suffering and make for a better existence so long as technology is constrained by moral principle. Without a firm grasp of moral principle and a knowledge of material and formal cooperation as it applies to new technologies, they cannot hope to persuade a secular pluralistic society in a way that makes legislative intervention a practical possibility.

More important than anything else, Catholics must function as a moral community which stands behind the human beings who must confront the choices and dilemmas that biological progress places before them. We must be prepared, as a Christian community shaped by the spirit of the Gospels, to assist those women contemplating abortion; to provide adoption services for those who, sadly, do not or cannot take care of their babies; to provide also for those handicapped infants who would have been deprived of treatment because the quality of their lives did not meet standards set by parents or society; to offer succor, pain relief and compassionate terminal care for the dying patients who might otherwise contemplate voluntary active euthanasia; to foster and facilitate adoption for sterile couples who might otherwise seek in vitro fertilization or surrogate motherhood.

We must also be able to distinguish legitimate research which does not violate moral principles from experimentation that does—between genetic manipulation, for example, that can correct inherited genetic diseases and manipulation aimed at eugenic improvement of the human species; between tissue transplants from spontaneous but not from electively aborted fetuses; and between fetal and embryo research aimed at benefits for the research subject and those without therapeutic benefit which result in the destruction of embryos.

Clearly, any attempt to shape legislation and civic law must depend upon influencing public opinion. This requires an informed Catholic community willing to engage in dialogue within its own membership and then with those outside the perimeters of its belief system. This dialogue is essential if we are to convince our fellow citizens that the issues with which *Donum Vitae* is concerned are moral, not political; that majority vote cannot make them morally valid; and that there are some acts, such as abortion and voluntary euthanasia, so morally grave that they cannot be left to private decision.

V. Recapitulation

Part III of *Donum Vitae* poses a serious challenge. It will be difficult to implement, given the moral trends so clearly visible in our society. Nonetheless, it is an obligation of Christians and Catholics to work to shape society so that at least the grosser moral assaults on human life are placed within constraints that are legal as well as moral. To fulfill this obligation, Catholics must confront the three dilemmas outlined here—the dilemmas of religious liberty, of consensual or majority vote ethics, and of influencing our democratic, secular, pluralistic society to enact laws that will conform to moral norms based in natural law as well as in revelation and ecclesiastical authority. This must be done within the framework of the procedures available to citizens of democratic societies and in a spirit that gives witness to the fundamental and central gospel message of charity.

Donum Vitae is far more than a disquisition on the morality of human procreation. It is a challenge to Catholics to live in such a way that the moral norms that should surround human procreation are made convincing by persuasion, dialogue, and personal behavior. This is nothing less than healing the rift between the temporal and the spiritual, not by military means or governmental fiat, but by democratic procedures, modulated by the gospel teachings of charity as the ordering principle of the Christian life.

Notes

1. Sacred Congregation for the Doctine of the Faith, "Instruction on Respect for Human Life in its Origin and on the Dignity of Procreation, Replies to Certain Questions of the Day" (Vatican City, 1986).

2. S. Taylor, Jr., "Catholic Tax Case to Get a Hearing," *New York Times*, 8 December 1987, A21.

3. K. A. Briggs, "Fight Abortion, O'Connor Urges Public Officials," *New York Times*, 16 October 1984, A1, B4; J. R. Dickenson, "Abortion Issue Draws Church Leaders into Presidential Push," *Washington Post*, 16 October 1984, A7.

4. Andrew M. Greeley, *Religious Change in America* (Cambridge, Mass.: Havard University Press, 1989).

5. *Roe v. Wade*, 410 U.S. 113 (1973).

6. *Reproductive Health Services v. Webster*, 662 F. Supp. 407 (W.D. Mo. 1987); 851 F.2d 1071 (8th Cir. 1988).

7. L. Greenhouse, "Abortion: Trouble Ahead, Three New Cases Will put Supreme Court on a Collision Course with *Roe v. Wade*," *New York Times*, 5 July 1989, A1.

174   Edmund D. Pellegrino

8. R. L. Risley and M. H. White, "Humane and Dignified Death Initiative for 1988," *The Euthanasia Review*, vol. 1, no. 4 (Winter 1986):226-39; Barbara Logue, *Death Control and the Elderly: The Growing Acceptability of Euthanisia* (Providence, R.I.: Brown University Population Studies and Training Center, April 1989; D. Humphrey and Ann Wickett, *The Right to Die: Understanding Euthanasia* (New York: Harper and Row, 1985).

9. *Report of the Human Fetal Tissue Transplantation Research Panel* (Washington, D.C.: U.S. Government Printing Office, December 1988).

10. American Fertility Society Ethics Committee, "Ethical Considerations of the New Reproductive Technologies," *Fertility and Sterility*, vol. 46 supplement (1986).

11. American Medical Association, Council on Ethical and Judicial Affairs, "Withholding or Withdrawing Life-Prolonging Medical Treatment," *JAMA* 256 (1986):471.

12. "Meeting of the Pontifical Academy of Sciences: Ethical, Medical and Legal Questions on the Artificial Prolongation of Life: Declaration Adopted by Scientists, *"L'Osservatore Romano*, 11 November 1965, 10; Catholic Bishops of New Jersey, "A Statement on the Sanctity of Life," *Origins*, vol. 14, no. 10 (9 August 1984).

13. John Lachs, "Active Euthanasia," unpublished paper presented at Summit Conference, Ottawa, Canada, 7 April 1988.

14. Mario Cuomo, "Religious Belief and Public Morality," *The Human Life Review*, vol. 11, nos. 1-2 (Winter-Spring 1985):26-40; S. Roberts, "Cuomo to Challenge Archbishop over Criticism of Abortion Stand," *New York Times*, 3 August 1984, A1, B2.

15. Morton White, *The Philosophy of the American Revolution* (New York: Oxford, 1981).

16. See especially *Dignitatis Humanae* and *Gaudium et Spes* in W. Abbott, ed., *The Documents of Vatican II* (London: Geoffrey Chapman, 1962); J. C. Murray, S.J., "The Issue of Church and State in Vatican II," *Theological Studies* 25 (1964):503-75.

17. National Conference of Catholic Bishops, "Catholic Social Teaching and the U.S. Economy: Health and Health Care: A Pastoral Letter of the American Catholic Bishops" (Washington, D.C.: U.S. Catholic Conference, 1981); "The Challenge of Peace: God's Promise and Our Response" (Washington, D.C.: U.S. Catholic Conference, 1983).

18. John Fletcher, "How Abortion Stifles Science," *Washington Post*, 5 February 1989.

19. B.J. Culliton, "Panel Backs Fetal Tissue Research," *Science* 242 (23 December 1988):1625.

20. Oxford English Dictionary, vol. 2 (Oxford: Clarendon Press, 1961), 850.

21. K.D. Clouser, "Allowing or Causing: Another Look," *Annals of Internal Medicine* 87 (1977):622-24; R.S. Dresser, J.D. and E.V. Boisaubin, Jr., M.D., "Ethics, Law and Nutritional Support," *Archives of Internal Medicine* 145 (1985):122-24; K.C. Micetich, P.H. Steinecker and D.C. Thomasma, "Are Intravenous Fluids Morally Required for a Dying Patient?," *Archives of Internal Medicine* 143 (1983):975-78; J. Lynn and J. Childress, "Must a Patient Always Be Given Food and Water?," *Hastings Center Report* 13 (1983):17-21.

22. I. Jakobovits, "Some Recent Jewish Views on Euthanasia," in D. Horan and D. Hall, eds., *Death, Dying and Euthanasia* (Washington, D.C.: University Publications, 1977), 344-47; Fred Rosner, *Modern Medicine and Jewish Law* (New York: Yeshiva University, 1972), 107-23.

23. E. D. Pellegrino, "Rationing Health Care: The Ethics of Medical Gatekeeping," *Journal of Contemporary Health Law and Policy* 2 (1986):23-45.

24. *In re Quinlan*, 70 N.J. 10, 355, A.2d 647, cert. denied 429 U.S. 922 (1976).

25. *In re Eichner*, 52 N.Y. 2d 363, 420 N.E. 2d 64, 438 N.Y.S. 2d 266, cert. denied, 454 U.S. 858 (1981).

26. *Barber v. Superior Court*, 147 Cal. App. 3d 1006, 195 Cal. Rptr. 484 (Ct. App. 1983).

27. *Bouvia v. Superior Court*, 179 Cal. App. 3d 1127, 225 Cal. Rptr. 297 (Ct. App.), review denied (5 June 1986).

28. *In re Infant Doe*, no. GU 8204-004A (Monroe County Circuit Ct., 12 April 1982).

29. *Weber v. Stony Brook, et. al.*, 467 N.Y.S. 2d 685.

30. *In re Baby M*, 13FLR 2001 (7 April 1987).

31. E. D. Pellegrino and V. A. Sharpe, "Medical Ethics in the Courts: The Need for Scrutiny," *Perspectives in Biology and Medicine* (Summer 1989).

32. See D. Horan, E.R. Grant and P.C. Cunningham, eds., *Abortion and the Constitution* (Washington, D.C.: Georgetown University Press, 1987).

33. See note 9, above.

34. See all reports of the President's Commission for the Study of Ethical Problems in Biomedical and Behavioral Research (Washington, D.C.: U.S. Government Printing Office, 1981-1983).

35. Alexander M. Capron, "Bioethics on the Congressional Agenda," *Hastings Center Report* (March/April 1989):22-23.

36. *Bouvia vs. Superior Court of Los Angeles County*, 179 Cal. App. 3d 1127, 225 Cal. Rptr. 297 (Ct. App.), review denied (5 June 1986), 307.

37. *In re Requena*, 517 A. 2d 886 (N.J. Super. Ch. Div. 1986), 517 A. 2d 869 (N.J. Super. 1986).

38. John Courtney Murray, S.J., *We Hold These Truths: Catholic Reflections on the American Proposition* (New York: Sheed and Ward, 1960).

39. Archbishop John R. Quinn, "*Donum Vitae* and Public Policy: Principles and Proposals," in this volume.

40. Thomas Aquinas, *Summa Theologiae*, (New York: Blackfriars, McGraw-Hill 1974), 2a2ae, Q. 91, art. 2; J.C. Murray, *We Hold These Truths*, 105.

41. Andrew Reck, "Natural Law and the Constitution," *Review of Metaphysics*, vol. 42, no. 3 (March, 1989):483-511.

42. J.C. Murray, *We Hold These Truths*, 333-34.

43. Ibid., 286.

44. John Locke, *Two Treatises of Government*, ed. Peter Laslett (Cambridge: Cambridge University Press, 1960).

45. Hugo Grotius, *On the Law of War and Peace*, trans. F.W. Kelsey (Oxford: Oxford University Press, 1986).

46. H.T. Engelhardt, Jr., *The Foundation of Bioethics* (New York: Oxford University Press, 1986).

47. Germain Grisez, "The Duty and Right to Follow One's Judgment of Conscience," *Linacre Quarterly* 56 (February, 1989):13-23.

ARCHBISHOP JOHN R. QUINN

Donum Vitae *and Public Policy:*
Principles and Proposals

My topic is the implications for public policy of the Instruction on Respect for Human Life in its Origin and on the Dignity of Procreation. In addressing this question, I speak as a bishop whose role it is both to teach the content of the document and represent its concerns in the public arena. The section of the Instruction which I will address is Part III entitled "Moral and Civil Law." This is the section of the Instruction which generated the most attention in the wider society.

Indeed, the amount and degree of attention paid to the Instruction indicate the concerns which exist in our society about the direction and implications of biomedical technology. Professionals as well as plain citizens have a mixed reaction: they marvel at the scientific advances, yet they question the social consequences which may flow from the new techniques. The concerns illustrate the validity of Dr. Daniel Callahan's comment that "the moral problems of biomedical ethics are beginning to transcend the narrow context of medicine itself. They are raising fundamental questions about how we ought to organize our society and think about our life together."[1] The social significance of medical technology is a theme which permeates the Instruction. It is precisely the social reach of the document which engages audiences beyond the Catholic Church. *The New York Times,* which featured four front-page stories on the document in eight days, welcomed it with an editorial which began: "On the day in 1978 that a little girl named Louise Brown was conceived in a Petri dish in a British laboratory, humankind took an enormous step into the future. Nine years later there is still no body of law to govern our residence there—nor are we really sure where to look for one."[2]

I will, then, discuss the social vision of the Instruction and its public policy positions in three steps: (1) a commentary on the Catholic style of argument in the Instruction; (2) an analysis of the principles it proposes to govern law and policy; and (3) a sketch of the relationship of these proposals to the United States public policy debate on bioethics.

1. The Catholic Style of Social Ethics and the Substance of the Instruction

The moral framework of the Instruction is an excellent example of a classical style of Catholic social ethics. Most of Catholic social teaching and much of Catholic medical ethics is grounded in natural law argument. The Instruction's moral case is a defense of the human person against unregulated technological intervention. The moral case is founded upon the natural moral law expressed in "rights and duties which are based upon the bodily and spiritual nature of the human person" (Intro. 3). The protection of human dignity through the defense of human rights is a persistent theme in the social teaching of this century, brought to its clearest articulation in *Peace on Earth* (1963) and John Paul II's address to the United Nations (1979). In the Instruction, this natural law social ethic is joined with a rejection of abortion and a defense of Catholic teaching on "the special nature of the transmission of human life in marriage" (Intro. 4). Both of these positions exemplify the natural law medical and sexual ethic. In fact, all the specific moral conclusions of the Instruction, e.g., the right to life of the fetus from conception, the criteria for prenatal diagnosis, the prohibition of in vitro fertilization (IVF), all flow—in a complex pattern—from the single structure of a natural ethic.

The character of the moral argument is directly linked to the public policy proposals of the document. The double purpose of using the natural law ethic in the Catholic tradition has been: (1) to provide a language and a structure for relating the moral wisdom derived from human reason and human experience to the moral vision of the Sacred Scriptures; and (2) to provide a theory of human values and basic moral principles in a mode which believers and others can use to formulate a moral position to address common problems.

The nature of the problems addressed in this Instruction engage the natural law ethic in both of its roles. On one hand, radically new choices which biotechnology makes possible require an extension—at times even a revision—of previously held conclusions in social and medical ethics. On the other hand, the problems or the possibilities inherent in these choices affect human society as a whole. As important as it is, an ecclesial or religious appeal will provide a response for part of society, but it may not evoke the kind of societal consensus needed to address the contemporary bioethical agenda.

The natural law character of the Instruction is revealed not only in the structure of the moral argument, but in the scope of its concerns. In the Instruction, equal attention is given to personal moral choice and to social policy or legislation affecting choice; in the perspective of this document sexual ethics are always seen in a social context. There is a strong rejection here of the notion that sexual and medical decisions about the beginning of life can be understood as purely "private choices," even though it is understood that they are deeply personal choices. The call for legislation in Part III flows directly and logically out of the moral framework of rights, duties and the social fabric of relationships which is found in Part I and Part II of the Instruction.

The classical philosophical structure of the Instruction roots it deeply in traditional Catholic social ethics; it also distinguishes it from the style of postconciliar social and moral teaching. This comparison of classical and contemporary social teaching is part of a larger theme. The shift from the perspective and language of *Peace on Earth* in 1963 to the content of the Pastoral Constitution *Gaudium et Spes* in 1965 is striking. The latter document, and much of the social teaching since then, uses a more explicitly biblical and theological argument, using categories which express the richness of Hebrew-Christian faith but which, for that very reason, have less utility in shaping a societal ethic for a pluralistic culture. The Instruction is more exclusively philosophical than the social teaching or the sexual ethic of John Paul II, which regularly incorporates biblical themes.

There is some blending of philosophical and theological themes in the argument made for the sacredness and inviolability of human life. A familiarity with the work of John Paul II would have led one to expect a more frequent use of the creation texts of Genesis which the Pope has used extensively in his encyclical *On Human Work* and in his discourses on sexuality and marriage. While the creation ethic of the Holy Father is not developed, another of his principal themes is highly visible: the relationship of technology and moral vision. On issues as disparate as medical-moral problems and nuclear weapons, the Pope reverts to the challenge of containing and directing technological developments within a structure of morally legitimated ends and morally acceptable means. The papal argument is never a case made against technological innovation, much less against the scientific research which is its foundation. A major concern of John Paul II is always that human control must be maintained over technology. The Instruction reflects this same concern in its warning that "one cannot derive criteria for guidance from mere technical efficiency," and in its axiom that "what is technically possible is not for that very reason morally admissible" (Intro. 2-4).

The essential argument of both the Pope and this Instruction is that technology should be submitted to political direction and politics should be guided by moral vision. One secular commentator described the Instruction as "a radical act of resistance to the technological hubris of modern reproductive medicine and to the Frankenstein world that it is rapidly making possible."[3] The starkness of this description points toward the difficulty of the task of ordering politics and technology by moral vision. The challenge of this task, and the consequences of failing in this effort, should be kept in mind as the Instruction is debated and evaluated in both church and society. The very scope of the Instruction, assessing both sexual practice and social legislation, guarantees that it will be a controversial document. But the strength and ultimate significance of the document more likely will derive from its broad social critique of trends in biomedical research and practice.

In this first section, I have tried simply to connect this contemporary social critique with a longer classical tradition of moral argument. The radical nature of the problems posed by biotechnologies can be personally disorienting and socially destabilizing. It is difficult to resist the notion that qualitative technological changes have cut us loose personally and collectively from the moral moorings which have guided medicine and politics for centuries. In this context, there is great value in a moral tradition which can relate the search for new answers to the structure of a moral argument based in a stable conception of human personality and the rights and duties which flow from such an anthropology.

2. The Principles of the Instruction and an Ethic for Public Policy

In its third part, the Instruction clearly declares that a purely personal ethic, relying only on a sense of responsibility and self-restraint in the medical profession and the research community, is an inadequate framework for the future. The nature of the problems posed by biotechnology requires "the intervention of the political authorities and of the legislator." The Instruction provides a guideline for this task: "The intervention of the public authority must be inspired by the rational principles which regulate the relationship between civil law and moral law." The source cited in the Instruction for these principles is the Declaration on Religious Liberty of Vatican II. Actually, the full range of questions posed by biotechnology goes beyond the principles found in the Declaration, but it points us in the right direction. The principal theological influence on the Declaration was, of course, Fr. John Courtney Murray, S.J. In his writings leading to the Vatican II document, Fr. Murray had explored the wider terrain of the role of civil law, its relationship to the moral law and its potential to direct the moral life of religiously pluralist societies.[4] Under the influence of Murray and others at Vatican II, the church amplified the traditional natural law conception of the relationship of state and society as well as the scope and function of civil law. I will summarize here the Instruction's reliance upon both the traditional elements of natural law and the developments produced by Vatican II.

The fundamental assertion of a natural law ethic is the requirement that the public life (civil law, public policy, professional practice) of a society be continually subjected to moral evaluation. It is this assertion which provides the foundation for the Instruction's "radical act of resistance" to technological innovation when it is not subject to moral evaluation. The fundamental assertion is a formal statement about the primacy of moral law as the foundation for civil order. The formal principle must be implemented through jurisprudential judgments and a process of casuistry. To move into this process of implementing the natural law assertion is to meet directly the question of the potential and the limits of civil law in the domain of biomedical problems. The Instruction clearly advocates the development of new laws to address new issues. But it manifests an awareness of the limits of civil law in its statement that the law "must sometimes tolerate, for the sake of public order, things which it cannot forbid without a greater evil resulting." How far can the civil law move in seeking to institutionalize moral principles in the life of society? Two realities set the framework for this question: the nature of civil law and the requirements of religious pluralism. I will deal with the question of civil law here, leaving comments on religious pluralism to the final section of this paper.

The civil law cannot and should not seek to embody the total scope of the moral law. Civil law has a more limited purpose; it seeks to regulate behavior affecting the external public order of society. Moral law encompasses a wider set of questions: thought and action; personal and public actions; dispositions and intentions. No human action falls beyond the scope of the moral law. Only certain categories of human actions fall within the competence of the civil law. Used within precise limits, the civil law complements the moral law by specifying and reinforcing key restraints on action. Used indiscriminately, the civil law can be extended into domains of personal life where its effect is counterproductive legally and even morally.

How to set proper limits for civil law, giving it space to function but recognizing its precise purpose? In an essay in 1960, Fr. Murray used three criteria to define the limits and the role of civil law.[5] First, the subject of the civil legislation must be an action with significant impact on the public order of society. The *public* consequences of the action to be prescribed or prohibited must be demonstrable. By definition, legislation imposes restraints or imposes responsibilities. Either of these consequences must be justified by the stake which society has in ensuring responsible activity by its citizens. This stress on the public implications of action means that some activities which would be judged morally wrong are not fit subjects for civil legislation if their public consequences are minimal.

Second, it if can be established that the activities in question do have substantial public consequences, the next test for civil law is whether a public consensus can be shaped to support passage and enforcement of the law. Failure to build a consensus risks exposing the authority of the law to disrespect, thereby threatening the institution of the law itself. The question of whether a social consensus must precede the imposition of civil law or whether reasonable legislation explained clearly and enforced equitably can build a consensus is a disputed topic in the United States. Some indeed invoke the lack of consensus about the morality and legality of abortion as a reason for not seeking more restrictive legislation. In their view, consensus should precede law. But others cite the example of civil rights legislation: both the Supreme Court decision of 1954 and the Civil Rights Act of 1964 were strongly opposed by significant sectors of the population. But law led the way toward civil consensus, changing American custom, habit and practice on race relations in the 1960s. A clear moral mandate for change had been recognized for decades, but the lack of civil legislation had impeded the process of translating the moral imperative into social policy. While differences continue to exist about the causal relationship of consensus and civil law, it is clear that the long-term viability of civil legislation requires a social consensus of support.

Third, to be beneficial to society, civil law must be enforceable in a way which does not impair or destroy values as significant as the ones the law is designed to protect or promote. This criterion requires an assessment of how a specific law fits into the wider structure of legislation and the broader fabric of the society. The Connecticut statute prohibiting the *use* by couples of contraception, which was struck down in the *Griswold* decision, was widely perceived to fail this third test. Even if a civil consensus against contraception did exist, enforcement of the law would have threatened other values of equal or greater significance.

These three criteria of jurisprudence have developed over time; they are a mix of moral principles, legal principles and the fruit of political experience. It is notable that in describing the role of civil law, the Instruction specifies its function in terms of serving the public order of society. The assimilation of the concept of public order, as Fr. Murray noted, is a product of recent developments in Catholic social teaching.[6] Since the idea of public order pertains directly to the first criterion for relating law and morality, there is a need to be precise about its content and applicability. The phrase "public order" appears for the first time in Catholic teaching in the Declaration on Religious Liberty (1965). Its purpose is to define the point at which the state has a right to restrict the exercise of the right of religious liberty. The formula used at Vatican II was that the state must show that a form of religious expression threatens the public order of society. While the term "public order" sounds both legalistic and even coercive, it has distinct moral content. Previous Catholic teaching often tied the state's role to the protection of the common good of society. The classical meaning of common good embodies a wide range of values. The common good is the total complex of spiritual and material conditions needed in society to create a setting in which human rights and duties may be fulfilled. If the scope of state action is defined as protecting the common good *in toto*, this provides an expansive role for coercive action and a potentially far-reaching role for civil law. Catholic social theory, with its strong organic conception of society, was inclined to favor a broad scope for both the role of the state and civil law.

The democratic revolutions of the eighteenth century, while stressing the value of freedom as an organizing principle for social life, were often godless and hostile to the church, and so did not find ready acceptance in nineteenth century Catholic teaching. But a dialogue was nevertheless set afoot about freedom which found a certain resolution in the Declaration on Religious Liberty. A major impetus in this dialogue was the experience of twentieth century totalitarianism. Without changing its basic position on the social nature of the person and organic order of society, Catholic teaching—led by Pius XII, John XXIII and Vatican II—came to a more positive conception of freedom and a somewhat more restrictive definition of the role of the state and civil law in society.

The more precise limits placed on state action become clear when the concept of the common good is contrasted with a definition of public order. Public order is comprised by three goods: public peace, public morality and protection of basic rights. To ensure these goods, it may be necessary to invoke the coercive power of the state. Hence the state is properly designated as the primary agent for the protection of public order, and civil law finds its primary role in specifying the needs of public order. The more expansive notion, the common good, is entrusted in recent Catholic teaching to the care of the whole society; other actors besides the state also have a responsibility for cultivating and protecting the values of the common good. The pertinence of this distinction for this paper is that it is conceivable that an action could be described as threatening to the common good but still not be a fit subject for legislation. It would only be appropriate to move toward civil law if a relationship to public order could be demonstrated. Indeed, the public order test is the first issue which must be resolved where the power of the state is to be invoked to restrain or command action.

If the three criteria for relating moral and civil law are used as a grid for assessing the legislative viability of positions taken in the Instruction, it is evident that a task of judgment and interpretation lies before us. The Instruction is clear in its moral conclusions and it is equally clear in its intent to have moral values protected by civil law in the biomedical field. But not all the moral conclusions of the Instruction move easily toward a legislative solution. Without trying to be comprehensive, I will sketch three different types of legislative judgment. The premise of this exercise is that I accept the moral conclusions of the Instruction; my sole concern is the feasibility of shaping "legislative intervention" as the Instruction describes it.

First, there are cases where the three criteria discussed above are met: public order is involved, consensus seems possible and enforcement does not sacrifice other values. Two examples found in the Instruction are surrogate mothers and nontherapeutic experimentation on embryos. While surrogacy is hotly debated,

186 John R. Quinn

the recent *Baby M* case has brought home forcefully the danger
of exploitation for many different parties to a surrogacy
contract—not least of these, the baby itself. Building consensus
around this issue seems possible and enforcement would not
violate a basic right of others. The Catholic position would find
other moral reasons in addition to exploitation to oppose
surrogacy, but the civil consensus could best be shaped in terms
of issues of justice. Nontherapeutic experimentation on embryos
is also a debated issue and ethical opinion in the United States
is not so clearly opposed to it as the Instruction is. But it does
raise serious issues of informed consent and subjecting the fetus
to unknown risks. Proving the public order case requires an
argument cast in terms of these two elements. Shaping a consensus may be more difficult on this issue; if such a consensus were
possible, equitable enforcement should also be possible.

Second, there are examples in the Instruction where the depth
and conviction of the church's opposition to an issue as well as
the inherent gravity of the issue means that as prophetic witness
and guardian of moral truth it must try for a legislative safeguard
of the values at stake, even though the chances of success may
be very slim. This is clearly the case in the Instruction's
opposition to abortion—opposing destruction of fetal life from
conception, and, therefore, opposing the destruction of "spare"
fertilized eggs in IVF. The drastic division in the United States
over abortion legislation makes implementation very difficult, even
though public order issues are clearly present here. The church
as prophetic defender of life and moral truth will be required to
press a legislative case even when the odds may be against success.

A third case would be examples where the church has a clear
moral position against an activity, but will not seek legislative
redress because public order concerns are not self-evident and
building a consensus is highly unlikely. The teaching in the
Instruction on homologous artificial insemination falls into this
category.

3. The Instruction and the U.S. Policy Debate

The cases just sketched illustrate the specifics of the policy debate. The detailed assessment of these examples would be a paper in itself. Rather than continue this microcosmic assessment of the policy process, the final section of this paper will relate the Instruction to the broad framework of the ethics and public policy discussion in the United States. Three themes are pertinent to this paper.

First, there is the character of the public discussion of ethics and social policy. The last fifteen years have witnessed an increasing role for moral argument in the U.S. public policy arena. The issues have been diverse: from nuclear strategy to human rights to civil rights to genetic research. These topics have always had a moral component, but the difference today is the explicit attention given to the moral dimension of policy. This attention is reflected in the literature for each field, in appeals made to morality during policy debates, and in the public interest generated by these topics. In many of these issues, failure to define a moral consensus can prove to be a major stumbling block to effective policy. While this general description of the morality and policy argument is significant, it is necessary to point out that of all the issues in the public debate the medical-moral questions have received the most thorough treatment. There is a serious, sustained tradition of analysis which has been developed in research institutes, in universities and under the auspices of four major governmental commissions. The details of the moral argument on experimentation, care of the terminally ill, abortion and genetics have been addressed more systematically than in any other area of public policy. This fact means that the Vatican Instruction fits into an ongoing field of research where it will join other well-established moral positions. The attention already paid to the document means that it will be part of the continuing debate, but it will not be used in isolation. Its conclusions and proposals are now part of a highly structured public agenda. The ability of the church to press for legislative action on these questions will depend heavily on the way its moral arguments are received.

Second, the ethics and public policy discussion takes place within a religiously pluralist society. The church in the United States must pursue all legislative goals within the requirements of pluralist dialogue. The religious voice has much freedom to speak and be heard, but the measure of its success is the ability to speak *from* a defined religious perspective *to* a pluralist constituency which can be persuaded by moral argument, but because of its pluralist make-up will not be commanded by religious authority. Fr. Murray argued that the only way for a religiously pluralistic society to avoid either constant conflict on the one hand or a moral vacuum on the other was to develop a core consensus of moral values and principles which could be held by believer and secularist, and by different communities of faith. The core consensus was simply an appeal to the notion of natural law. The case Murray made for this public ethic was that certain issues in society were too central in their importance and too pervasive in their consequences to be left to a series of private, individual choices.[7] On some questions, the society as a whole had to set a moral direction for action. The advent of biomedical advances came after Murray's death but they illustrate his theme with new urgency. The shaping of the core consensus is a delicate and difficult task, but it is the precondition to finding adequate response of law and policy in the area of bioethics.

Third, in the religiously pluralist conversation which must shape any consensus, the church must see itself as one actor in a complex matrix of institutions. The new visibility of ethical themes in the public debate has not been solely or—in the biomedical field—even principally the product of religious insight. Universities and research institutes have been the major catalysts in the biomedical debate: philosophers and lawyers, physicians and scientists all are key actors in the moral debate.

In the United States, the relationship between the moral law and civil law has several forums. To shape a consensus on biomedical issues means addressing both federal and state legislation. But it also means appreciating the distinct and powerful role of the courts where much of contemporary decision making in bioethics is carried on. The Vatican document inevitably must state its case in general terms; in calling for the intervention of political authorities and legislators, it has touched a highly complex agenda in the United States. The church here cannot remain at the general level of the Instruction. It must proceed with political sophistication, moral sensitivity and ecumenical tact if it is to enter the law and policy debate effectively.

Notes

1. D. Callahan, "The Hastings Center: Ethics in the 1980's," *Hastings Center Report* 11(1981):1-2 (supp.).

2. *New York Times*, 11 March 1987, A1.

3. C. Krauthammer, "The Ethics of Human Manufacture," *New Republic* (4 May 1987), 17.

4. J.C. Murray, *We Hold These Truths* (New York: Sheed and Ward, 1960); J.C. Murray, "The Problem of Religious Freedom," *Theological Studies* 25(1964):503-75.

5. Murray, *We Hold These Truths*, 155-74.

6. Murray, "The Problem of Religious Freedom," 529-30.

7. Murray, *We Hold These Truths*, 27ff. and 79ff.

STEVEN P. FRANKINO, J.D.

The Legal Limits of Donum Vitae

The Vatican Instruction in its third part, "Moral Law and Civil Law," addresses legal considerations and political implementation of its teachings. In doing so, it reads in the traditional language of Judeo-Christian natural law jurisprudence. A fundamental problem concerning the relevancy of the Instruction is that it limits the legal context to systems which are derived from Roman law and canon law. Thus it speaks with some clarity to the Western European political and legal tradition and limits its impact for that very reason. There is no recognition of other major legal systems such as Anglo-American common law, socialist law, or Islamic law. The first and second parts of the Instruction are based on general scientific and medical knowledge and practice and universal moral and theological considerations, yet the practical impact in the secular sphere is narrowed because it is based on legal and political assumptions which are not applicable in some of the most important areas of the church's mission. Legal and political experts from other traditions should have been consulted so that the Instruction could inform social and political action beyond the sphere of Western European continental jurisprudence.

An example of this misplaced legal analysis can be found in the identification of national and local authorities to which the Instruction is addressed. It presumes that political authorities are the source of law and legal implementation. Thus it addresses the obligations of executive and administrative bodies and legislative assemblies. These governmental functions are the primary sources of law in unitary states and European parliamentary states. In those states, the judicial function has little or no policy-making role. Yet in common law countries, the judicial function is of significance in the definition, interpretation and implementation of legal norms. In the United States, and in those nations which have followed the American constitutional approach such as Ireland, the judiciary has a separate role in addressing the legal issues encompassed in the Instruction. For this reason, the Instruction presents major difficulties in translation to common jurisdictions and particularly to a constitutional jurisprudence which articulates a secular natural law.

The assumption of the Instruction is that the competent authority for the protection of rights is the legislator and that the competent enforcer is the executive or administrative political authority. This assumption is not valid in the context of United States constitutional law. Most of the issues in science, medicine and ethics covered by the Instruction will be given their final definition and application by courts. An important policy maker in most of these areas will be the United States Supreme Court.

It should be noted that the Instruction creates similar difficulties in relation to the development of national and transnational judicial decision making in both Europe and Latin America. The Constitutional Courts of Germany and Italy are developing policy-making roles. In addition, the Courts of Human Rights established by European and Latin American international conventions are developing an important body of judicial decisions with potential application to the subject matter of the Instruction.

Having noted the serious limitations placed on the relevancy of Part III of the Instruction because of its narrowed civil law perspective, I will illustrate these legal difficulties in the context of the law of the United States. In approaching these legal issues, a distinction must be made between the Judeo-Christian natural law tradition and the secular natural law as found and applied in American courts, particularly in the United States Supreme Court. The pervasive value in American jurisprudence is personal liberty or freedom.[1] From this is derived the protected nature of family decisions.[2] Rights found in United States secular natural law protecting the autonomy of familial judgments are the right to determine the place, content and context of children's education;[3] the right to privacy within the marital status,[4] including the right to have access to contraceptives;[5] the right to privacy in the decision whether to bear or beget a child,[6] a right applicable to the individual whether married or single;[7] and the correlative right to procreate.[8] The nature of the rights found and articulated by the courts is based on the freedom of the individual from unwarranted governmental interference with procreative capabilities.[9] The definition of these personal liberties determines the permissible scope of legislation.[10]

The Vatican Instruction presumes that political power exists which will be competent to fashion legislation in relation to procreative matters. This is correct to a marked degree in relation to European and Third World nations. In the American context, the political branches of state and federal governments cannot enact statutes and regulations free from constitutional scrutiny by the Supreme Court. The political power is limited by the secular natural law jurisprudence of the judicial branch.

In the American context there are only two means for changing the jurisprudence of individual rights based upon liberty in the family and procreative areas: (1) a dramatic fundamental change in the jurisprudence of the United States Supreme Court reexamining and reversing hundreds of cases which reach back more than a century, or (2) amending the Constitution. When the Instruction addresses the obligations of persons within the American polity to implement the moral and theological norms set forth, there is basic misunderstanding of the legal reality of the United States. There is a conflict of values when the formulations of the Instruction are set off against the rights articulated in American constitutional law.

The values articulated by the United States Supreme Court are rights of individual or personal liberty while the Instruction teaches the right to life and physical integrity. The right to privacy within marriage is set off against the right of the family. The right of privacy of the individual, whether married or single, in the decision to bear or beget a child is in contradiction to the Instruction's rights of the institution of marriage. Finally, the constitutional right of the individual to procreate or not to procreate is set off against the child's right to be conceived and the dignity of procreation. In sum, there is a fundamental value conflict between the jurisprudence of the United States Supreme Court and the teachings of the Holy See.

Because of this fundamental disagreement concerning civic values and the content of moral law, there will be only limited areas for congruence in the application of law. Insofar as the Instruction calls for the intervention of political authorities and of legislation and, as Archbishop Quinn has stated, the Instruction "clearly advocates the development of new laws to address new issues," there are substantial constitutional limitations in the United States to the implementation of the Holy See's goals. Legislation restricting access to abortion[11] or to contraception[12] would not pass constitutional muster. The same conclusion would most likely apply to legal attempts to restrict in vitro fertilization and embryo transplant for procreative purposes.[13] Both would seem to be well within the ambit of the protected right to procreate. Any attempted legislation involving these issues would be subject to strict judicial scrutiny.[14]

Very different legal considerations are involved in regard to nontherapeutic experimentation on embryos and the destruction of in vitro fertilized eggs.[15] The family and individual rights articulated in procreative issues would not have application in the area of nontherapeutic experimentation. The legislature should be free to fashion statutes forbidding or restricting such procedures. As Archbishop Quinn has noted, political consensus seems possible in this area. In fact, both state and federal laws and regulations have already addressed the issues.

Since 1973, regulation of experimentation has been moving forward on both the national and state levels.[16] The federal government has placed restrictions on fetal experimentation through its power to regulate those who receive funding for research. The Department of Health and Human Services and the National Institutes of Health have promulgated regulations concerning both therapeutic and nontherapeutic experimentation.[17]

During the same period of time the legislatures of more than half the states have passed statutes regulating fetal experimentation. In addition, all states have passed the Uniform Anatomical Gift Act, which governs experimentation on dead fetuses.[18] The Act includes within the definition of "decedent" any "stillborn infant or fetus." Although state statutes beyond the limited scope of the Uniform Act are anything but uniform, a majority of states which have legislation have prohibited nontherapeutic experimentation on live aborted fetuses. This is an area in which there can be a congruence of goals of the civil and moral law. Archbishop Quinn has noted that experimentation is an area where the moral force of the Instruction and the influence of the church can have significant impact on the adoption and implementation of statutes.

It should be noted that the experimentation issue is not completely free from possible constitutional limitation, in particular in the setting of colleges and universities, including teaching and research medical facilities. There are legal developments which articulate a First Amendment free speech interest in pure scientific research. It is early to predict what the final determination of this issue might be. There are liberty interests in the development and free flow of ideas. Access to and promulgation of knowledge has been recognized as a value within the First Amendment's freedoms. However, these values are subject to reasonable legislative restriction and limitation.

The final issues addressed by Archbishop Quinn relate to surrogate motherhood. He suggested that this is an area in which "public order is involved," and "consensus seems possible and enforcement does not sacrifice other values." Of all of the matters addressed in the Instruction, surrogacy raises the most complex legal considerations.[19] In fact, a separate conference could fruitfully explore the interdisciplinary and legal aspects of surrogate motherhood. There are overreaching legal issues affecting the status of surrogate motherhood as an expression of, or as an affront to, basic civic and moral values. This is especially true in regard to family recognition, structure and function. In addition to these fundamental concerns, there are issues which are common to a number of artificial conception techniques. Among these is the parental status of gamete donors. Other issues are peculiar to a particular technology, such as whether the flushing of an ovum fertilized *in vivo* constitutes an abortion.

Legislative responses to surrogate motherhood are already in place. Half of the states have statutes regulating artificial insemination.[20] Surrogate contracts have been prohibited directly or indirectly. Where the surrogate contract is allowed, the permissible terms of the contract must be examined. For example, can the contract forbid the surrogate from using alcohol or tobacco, compel amniocentesis, require an abortion, or prevent an abortion? Can the surrogate sue for payment under the contract; sue for expenses; sue for child support or place an unwanted child in adoption? Can a court specifically enforce the contract against the adopting couple to obligate them to accept an unwanted child? Is the surrogate contract a violation of constitutional provisions prohibiting ownership or trade and commerce in human beings? The legal issues are almost without end. What is clear is that surrogate motherhood involves all of the philosophical, theological and legal considerations set forth in the Vatican Instruction.

I will close my observations concerning Part III of the Instruction where I began—with the United States Supreme Court. In the initial decision concerning the right of privacy in abortion, *Roe v. Wade*, the Court wrote: "When those trained in the respective disciplines of medicine, philosophy, and theology are unable to arrive at any consensus, the judiciary, at this point in the development of man's knowledge, is not in a position to speculate as to the answer."[21] The "consensus" which the Court was referring to is the unanswered question of when life begins. This question "may present an insurmountable hurdle to the legal world in defining the rights and duties of the unborn child, its parents, and the scientists responsible for its creation."[22] As long as that consensus is absent from the pluralistic society of the United States, much of the subject matter covered in the Instruction will be outside of the public consensus requirement articulated by Father John Courtney Murray's criteria as set forth and applied by Archbishop Quinn in his paper. Even though the intrinsic significance of issues such as abortion means that the church must strive for legislative safeguards, the problem for the Catholic lay person as a legislator, executive or judge is not answered. Since the Instruction gives very limited guidance to those who live in secular pluralistic common law societies, there is little instruction or comfort for those who labor in the civil vineyard. I personally find this failure of the Instruction to be not only disappointing but frustrating. Political and legal professionals in the United States must look elsewhere for help in facing the moral dilemmas often confronted in service to Caesar and to God.[23]

Notes

1. *Palko v. Connecticut*, 302 U.S. 319 (1937). The U.S. Supreme Court recognized personal rights "implicit in the concept of ordered liberty" so fundamental that they are an independent source of constitutional protection (325). In *Roe v. Wade*, 410 U.S. 113, 152 (1973), the Court found a woman's privacy rights in the decision to have an abortion to be within the protection of the Fourteenth Amendment.

2. *Meyer v. Nebraska*, 262 U.S. 390 (1923); *Pierce v. Society of Sisters*, 268 U.S. 510 (1925).

3. Robertson, "Procreative Liberty and the Control of Conception, Pregnancy and Childbirth," *Virginia Law Review* 69 (1983):405.

4. *Griswold v. Connecticut*, 381 U.S. 479 (1965) (a state statute which prohibited the use of contraceptives was struck down because the statute violated the right of marital privacy which was found to be protected by the Constitution).

5. *Carey v. Population Serv. Int'l.*, 431 U.S. 678 (1977) (a state statute which restricted the distribution, sale, advertising and display of contraceptives was struck down). "Read in the light of its progeny, the teaching of *Griswold* is that the Constitution protects individual decisions in matters of childbearing from unjustified intrusion by the State... This is so not because there is an independent fundamental 'right to contraceptives,' but because such access is essential to exercise of the constitutionally protected right of decision in matters of childbearing that is the underlying foundation of the holdings in *Griswold, Eisenstadt v. Baird*, and *Roe v. Wade*," 687-89.

6. Ibid, p. 686. The Court held that if a regulation infringes upon a constitutionally protected fundamental right, the state must show a "compelling" interest. "'Compelling' is of course the key word; where a decision as fundamental as that whether to bear or beget a child is involved, regulations imposing a burden on it may be justified only by compelling state interests, and must be narrowly drawn to express only those interests."

7. *Eisenstadt v. Baird*, 405 U.S. 438 (1972) (a statute which prevented distribution of contraceptives to single but not married persons was found to be unconstitutional). "If the right of privacy means anything, it is the right of the *individual* married or single, to be free from unwarranted governmental intrusion into matters so fundamentally affecting a person as the decision whether to bear or beget a child," 453 (emphasis in the original).

8. *Skinner v. Oklahoma*, 316 U.S. 535 (1942) (a state statute which permitted sterilization of criminals under certain circumstances was held to be unconstitutional). "We are dealing here with legislation which involves one of the basic civil rights of man. Marriage and procreation are fundamental to the very existence and survival of the race," 541.

9. Ibid.

10. *San Antonio School District v. Rodriguez*, 411 U.S. 1 (1973).

11. *Roe v. Wade*, 410 U.S. 113 (1973); *City of Akron v. Akron Center of Reproductive Health*, 462 U.S. 416 (1983).

12. *Griswold v. Connecticut*, 381 U.S. 479 (1965); *Eisenstadt v. Baird*, 405 U.S. 438 (1972); *Carey v. Population Serv. Int'l.*, 431 U.S. 678 (1977).

13. Williams, "Legislative Guidelines to Govern In Vitro Fertilization and Embryo Transfer," *Santa Clara Law Review* 26 (1986):495; Fanta, "Legal Issues Raised by In Vitro Fertilization and Embryo Transfer in the United States," *Journal of In Vitro Fertilization and Embryo Transfer* 2 (1985):65; Andrews, "The Legal Status of the Embryo," *Loyola Law Review* 32 (1986):357.

14. See Williams, "Legislative Guidelines," 514.

15. "Tempest in the Laboratory: Medical Research on Spare Embryos from In Vitro Fertilization," *Hastings Law Journal* 37 (1986):977; G. Smith, "Australia's Frozen 'Orphan' Embryos: A Medical, Legal and Ethical Dilemma," *Journal of Family Law* 24 (1985):27.

16. Armstrong, "Womb and Board: Medical Advances in Reproduction—At What Cost?" *Medical Trial Technique Quarterly* 33 (1987):466.

17. National Research Act, Public Law no. 92-348, §213, 88 Stat. 353 (1974); 42 U.S.C. §2891-1; 40 FR 33528, 8 August 1975 as amended at 4FR 51638, 6 November 1975; 45 C.F.R. §§46.201-46.211.

18. "Uniform Anatomical Gift Act," 8A *Unif. Laws Annotated* 8A:15-16 (1983).

19. Stumf, "Redefining Mother: A Legal Matrix for New Reproductive Technologies," *Yale Law Journal* 96 (1986):187.

20. Shapiro, "New Innovations in Conception and Their Effects upon Law and Morality," *New York Law School Law Review* 31 (1986):37 and 42.

21. *Roe v. Wade*, 159.

22. Shapiro, "New Innovations," 39.

23. M. Cuomo, "Religious Belief and Public Morality: A Catholic Governor's Perspective," *Journal of Law, Ethics and Public Policy* 1 (1984):13.